A
FIRST
GROUP
PSYCHOTHERAPY
BOOK

A FIRST GROUP PSYCHOTHERAPY BOOK

By
EDWARD L. PINNEY, Jr., M.D.

With a Foreword by
AARON STEIN, M.D.

JASON ARONSON INC.
Northvale, New Jersey
London

THE MASTER WORK SERIES

First softcover edition 1995

Library of Congress Cataloging-in-Publication Data

Pinney, Edward Lowell, 1925–
    A first group psychotherapy book / by Edward L. Pinney, Jr.
      p.   cm.
    Originally published: Springfield, Ill. : C.C. Thomas, 1970.
    Includes bibliographical references and index.
    ISBN 1-56821-617-3
    1. Group psychotherapy.   2. Group psychotherapy—Case studies.
I. Title.
RC488.P55   1995
616.89′152—dc20

95-17203

FOREWORD

In this book, Dr. Pinney has given a concise, clear, and straightforward exposition of the basic elements in group psychotherapy. In addition to the clarity of his description of the dynamic factors in this form of treatment, he has selected portions of tape-recorded, verbatim transcripts of group sessions which vividly illustrate the working of group psychotherapy. These provide a vividness of detail that brings to life, so to speak, the interaction and dynamic interplay of the patients in the group and the group therapist.

This, then, is truly a "first group psychotherapy book"—a book which states clearly and simply the basic dynamics of group psychotherapy. The limitations and usefulness of this form of treatment are also succinctly and honestly stated, a most desirable statement when compared with the exaggerated claims being put forth for many forms of group treatment.

Dr. Pinney is also quite precise in indicating that his theoretical concepts concerning the dynamics of group psychotherapy, while utilizing psychoanalytic concepts and terminology, encompass what might be called a more eclectic viewpoint. He feels that many of the characteristic ways in which an individual functions—his character, personality, and particularly his ego structure—are "socially determined (often family determined)." They are the result of "systems of adaptation" stemming from social influences. Therefore, according to Dr. Pinney, the patient's "style of mental functioning . . . can be examined in the group psychotherapy and the social pressure of the group can serve to reshape" these characteristic social patterns and "offer new ways of managing inner forces and interpersonal relationships."

Based on these concepts, Dr. Pinney gives a concise and very clear description of the kind of patient who is most suitable for group psychotherapy. On the whole, those patients who have moderate to severe illness are most suitable, according to Dr. Pinney, and in general, most workers would agree in this respect.

How such severely ill patients are helped by group psychotherapy is graphically illustrated in the transcripts of the group sessions. The discussion of ways in which patients are selected for participation in the group and the various factors to be considered is most useful.

In the second chapter, Dr. Pinney offers an interesting discussion of the training of the group therapist. He describes a method he has used for some time with good results. What is most illuminating here are his remarks about the limitations some psychotherapists have which tend to interfere with their ability to do group psychotherapy.

Different types of groups are described, and the important point is made that the kind of patient and the setting both determine the kind of group psychotherapy that is utilized.

Following this, Dr. Pinney describes the first meetings of a newly formed group, illustrated by selections from transcripts of group sessions. He then discusses the patient's reaction to the first group session, pointing out clearly the nature of the anxiety, the defensive reactions, and the transference attitudes that the patient will experience and how these need to be brought out and handled.

His discussion of the task of the group therapist is thorough, clear, and most useful. The timing of interventions and interpretations, the handling of resistances, and the manner in which these are to be made are gone into in detail, as are cautions against faulty technique. What constitutes improvement and the goal toward which the group therapist should work is discussed in a straightforward, workmanlike manner, and the limitations are indicated in this form of treatment with rather severely ill patients.

The way in which the work of the group and the therapist is carried out is described with clarity and is beautifully illustrated in a series of verbatim excerpts from two groups. Here, all the dynamics are evident: identification, universalization, projection, etc. How these are used to deny and resist are clearly demonstrated, and how discussions can be guided by the therapist to overcome resistance and to bring out problems and conflicts with their attendant emotions are ably demonstrated. The material is most interesting and made eminently clear by Dr. Pinney's concise and apt comments.

The manner in which Dr. Pinney demonstrates group interaction through excerpts from the group sessions and the way in which the patients and the therapist function in group psychotherapy may be considered the most enlightening and valuable features of this book. The skill with which the excerpts were chosen and the concise, understandable fashion in which the important points were made represent a major achievement. Together, they make this a very valuable "first group psychotherapy book" in teaching and demonstrating the basic principles of group psychotherapy. Dr. Pinney is to be highly commended for contributing a much-needed addition to the teaching literature of group psychotherapy.

AARON STEIN

INTRODUCTION

This book provides instructions for psychotherapists who want to do group psychotherapy, a theoretical basis for group psychotherapy, and transcriptions of the discussions at group psychotherapy sessions as illustrations of techniques for study.

At this time, no other book provides these features. The need for some direction for the beginner is apparent.

The theoretical basis for group psychotherapy provided in this book has been derived from experience and the theories of mental function available. This theoretical basis is correlated with the selection of patients for group psychotherapy and has influenced the selection of the verbatim excerpts from group psychotherapy discussions provided in the text.

The main features, the fundamentals, of group psychotherapy are included. Unproven, controversial, and nonessential matters have been excluded in the interest of directness and utility. The fundamentals are presented in a style aimed at providing practical information.

In my experience, group psychotherapy is better suited for the sicker patients and consequently my theoretical formulation is different from those who feel that group psychotherapy closely resembles psychoanalysis. I have included verbatim reports on group psychotherapy sessions to illustrate my approach.

Dr. George Naumberg, Jr., introduced me to group psychotherapy when I was a student in medical school. I was working at the Northport, New York, Veterans Administration Hospital during the summer of 1948 when he permitted me to sit with his group of severely disturbed patients, most of whom were suicidal and homicidal chronic catatonic schizophrenics. In the group they discussed their symptoms and talked with one another. On returning to the ward, many of the patients resumed a stuporous attitude. The dramatic response of these patients to group psychotherapy was impressive.

Later that year, while a medical student in St. Louis, I audited some of Dr. Nathan Blackman's group psychotherapy training sessions at the Malcolm A. Bliss Psychopathic Institute, the psychiatric division of St. Louis City Hospital.

At the Brooklyn State Hospital from 1952 to 1955, Dr. J. J. Lawton's training program in group psychotherapy under the direction of Dr. Nathan Beckenstein provided me with supervisional experience in group psychotherapy. One result of this work was my preparation of a paper entitled "The Use of Recorded Minutes in Group Psychotherapy: A Preliminary Report on a New Technique"* and of another on "Reactions of Outpatient Schizophrenics to Group Psychotherapy."†

Subsequently, I engaged in private practice with outpatient groups. This led to the publication of two additional papers that I wrote: "The Use of Recorded Minutes in Group Psychotherapy: The Development of a 'Readback' Technique"‡ in 1963, and "The Psychiatric Indications for Group Psychotherapy"§ in 1965.

I have continued doing group psychotherapy in my private practice. It has worked out well as the treatment of choice for certain types of patients.

My work in teaching psychiatric residents at the Kings County Hospital Center Psychiatric Hospital Group Psychotherapy Training Program of the State University of New York Downstate Medical Center from 1964 through 1967 has provided the opportunity for much thought provoking discussion. Dr. Abbott Lippman headed this teaching program.

At the beginning of 1968, I began the teaching of group psychotherapy at the Cornell University Medical College training program for psychiatry residents at the Payne Whitney Division of The New York Hospital.

---

* Pinney, E. L., Jr.: The use of recorded minutes in group psychotherapy: A preliminary report on a new technique. *Psychiat. Quart.* [*Supp*], Pt. 2, 1955.

† Pinney, E. L., Jr.: Reactions of outpatient schizophrenics to group psychotherapy. *Int. J. Group Psychother.*, Vol. VI, April, 1956, No. 2.

‡ Pinney, E. L., Jr.: The use of recorded minutes in group psychotherapy: The development of a "readback" technique. *Psychiat. Quart.* [*Supp*], Pt. 2, 1963.

§ Pinney, E. L., Jr.: The psychiatric indications for group psychotherapy. *Psychosomatics,* Vol. VI, May-June, 1965, pp. 139–144.

I have been fortunate in being able to participate in panel discussions on group psychotherapy at the annual meetings of the American Psychiatric Association in 1965, 1966, 1967, 1968 and 1969* with Dr. Donald A. Shaskan, Dr. Aaron Stein, Dr. Clifford J. Sager and Dr. Hyman Spotnitz. These discussions and the personal communications from these panelists have been among the most intellectually stimulating experiences I have encountered.

Many others, for instance, Dr. Thomas Thale and Dr. Warren B. Mills in St. Louis, have been encouraging and helpful. Dr. Jan Frank and several others have contributed toward the development of my ideas during the last twenty years.

I would like to express my thanks to Miss Phyllis Cohen and Mr. Albert Sherman for their services in preparation of the manuscript for this book and to Mr. Hyman Sandow, who has been of invaluable editorial help.

New York City   EDWARD L. PINNEY, JR.

* Group Psychotherapy Is Indicated for Severely Ill Patients Who Have Some Tolerance for Their Psychopathology. Shaskan, D. A., Moderator; Pinney, E. L., Jr., Secretary; Sager, C. J.; Spotnitz, H.; Stein, A.: *Scientific Proceedings in Summary Form.* The One Hundred and Twenty-first Annual Meeting of the American Psychiatric Association, 1965, p. 334.

The Mechanisms of Group Psychotherapy: Insight or Feedback? (The same panelists.) *Scientific Proceedings in Summary Form.* The One Hundred and Twenty-second Annual Meeting of the American Psychiatric Association, 1966, p. 289.

The Mechanisms of Group Psychotherapy: The Results of Group Pressure. (The same panelists.) *Scientific Proceedings in Summary Form.* The One Hundred and Twenty-third Annual Meeting of the American Psychiatric Association, 1967, p. 309.

The Mechanisms of Group Psychotherapy: Achieving the Therapists' Goal. (The same panelists.) *Scientific Proceedings in Summary Form.* The One Hundred and Twenty-fourth Annual Meeting of the American Psychiatric Association, 1968, p. 350.

What's Therapeutic "Activity" in Group Therapy. (The same panelists.) *Scientific Proceedings in Summary Form.* The One Hundred and Twenty-fifth Annual Meeting of the American Psychiatric Association, 1969, p. 297.

CONTENTS

A FIRST GROUP PSYCHOTHERAPY BOOK

Chapter 1

HISTORICAL BACKGROUND

The ancient Greek dramatists may be said to have been group psychotherapists if one believes that catharsis is the main feature of group psychotherapy. Aristotle, in his *Poetics*, refers to catharsis as a mental mechanism for the audience at plays. The phenomena of group psychotherapy, however, include far more than catharsis and provide more specific mechanisms for the resolution of the problems of each patient in a psychotherapy group.

Group psychotherapy began with the work of Dr. Joseph Henry Pratt in 1905. A Boston internist, Dr. Pratt developed a plan for the treatment of consumption in the homes of patients. He called the group a "tuberculosis class." These classes consisted of fifteen to twenty patients who met once a week. The results in Dr. Pratt's classes were favorable; other physicians who tried to follow his example were not nearly so successful. Pratt's personality appears to have been so constructed that he carried out his work intuitively. The improvement in the emotional state of patients in Pratt's classes led to the use of this treatment method for patients suffering from mental disorders.

Dr. Elwood Worchester, Director of the Emmanuel Church in Boston, advanced money to Pratt to help him start his tuberculosis classes. Later, Dr. Worchester, aided by Isidore Coriat, one of the first members of the American Psychoanalytic Association, began seeing patients in groups to assist them with their health problems. These groups were not limited to tuberculosis patients.

Pratt independently continued his interest in group treatment, but shifted his attention to patients with emotional problems. It must be noted that no theoretical basis for group psychotherapy that could be used in teaching this technique nor carrying out worthwhile research had yet appeared. Pratt eventually applied the ideas of Joseph Deperine, which emphasized persuasion and reeducation. Pratt continued his work as a group psychotherapist into the 1950's.

Psychiatric patients, as such, were treated by group psychotherapy as early as 1921, when Lazelle treated schizophrenics in this way. Lazelle had been preceded in 1909 by Marsh, who had worked with groups of psychotics in classes and lectures. Marsh's groups probably would not be recognizable as psychotherapy groups; however, he recognized the therapeutic value of group activities for psychotics.

Patients in another category, institutionalized borderline cases, were treated by Louis Wender in the late 1920's and early 1930's. Wender spoke of his groups as being "psychoanalytic" rather than "educational and orientation," as he viewed the others. Wender saw six to eight patients in each group, two or three times a week. The groups were of the same sex and each session lasted one hour. He combined individual and group psychotherapy and suggested that the group might represent the family to the patient. Paul Schilder at Bellevue also worked with groups in which he used "psychoanalytic" techniques.

The term "group psychotherapy" is said to have been first used by J. L. Moreno. In any case, he was one of the first to use it.* He is the leading exponent of psychodrama, a treatment technique related to group psychotherapy.

In the 1930's Samuel Slavson, a civil engineer, practiced activity group psychotherapy with children for the Jewish Board of Guardians. His book, *An Introduction to Group Therapy*, was published in 1943.† Subsequently, Slavson was instrumental in the formation and development of the American Group Psychotherapy Association. In 1951 he became the first editor of the *International Journal of Group Psychotherapy*. Slavson has written several other books and has played an active role in the advancement of group psychotherapy as a force in psychiatry and social work.

---

* Moreno, J. L.: *Group Psychotherapy—A Symposium.* New York, Beacon House, 1945, p. 18.

† Slavson, S. R.: *An Introduction to Group Therapy.* New York, Commonwealth Fund, 1943.

Group psychotherapy was one of the many new techniques that were more extensively utilized in the great development and expansion of medical treatment methods that began during the late 1930's and continued to grow explosively throughout World War II and into the postwar period.

The influence of psychoanalysis on psychiatry in the United States was evident in the late 1930's and became more prominent during World War II and the subsequent years. During this period, theoretical formulations based on psychoanalysis and intensive individual psychotherapy were applied to group psychotherapy.

During World War II group psychotherapy had begun to be practiced extensively in military hospitals. After the war psychiatrists returning to civilian practice took their treatment technique with them and applied it in nonmilitary settings.

S. H. Foulkes, a British psychoanalyst, contributed greatly to the literature on group psychotherapy. He started his work as a group psychotherapist with military personnel during World War II and continued to practice group psychotherapy during the postwar period. His book, *Introduction to Group Analytic Psychotherapy*, appeared in 1949.*

In the United States, Alexander Wolf described his techniques and therapeutic approaches in articles in the *American Journal of Psychotherapy* in 1949 and 1950.†

Foulkes and Wolf are the originators of the group psychotherapy we know today. They spoke of group psychotherapy as an independent entity with a rationale and a discipline all its own. Wolf, in particular, described techniques that are fundamental to this treatment method.

Foulkes and Wolf applied psychoanalytic formulations to groups of patients. Wolf spoke of the psychoanalysis of groups and Foulkes has applied the psychoanalytic resolution of transferences to group psychotherapy.

---

* Foulkes, S. H.: *Introduction to Group Analytic Psychotherapy*. New York, Grune, 1949.

† Wolf, Alexander: The psychoanalysis of groups. *Amer. J. Psychother.*, Vol. III, No. 4, October, 1949; Vol. IV, No. 1, January, 1950.

The time has come to utilize formulations for group psychotherapy that do not directly follow the one-to-one treatment phenomena of psychoanalysis. The direct comparison of individual psychoanalysis with group psychotherapy can be useful in understanding certain phenomena in the interaction in the group psychotherapy. However, other formulations based on the relationship between development of the style of the ego or character, which is socially determined, are more appropriate and represent the new phase in the understanding of the phenomena of group psychotherapy.

The interaction between patients in the group and the relation of the leader to the group have some relevance to Freud's thinking on group psychology.* The psychoanalytic formulations relating to the social influences on the systems of adaptation referred to as "character" provide a basis for the development of therapeutic formulations about group psychotherapy.† The microsociety of the group can help the individual understand his activity elsewhere. The adaptive patterns acceptable to and possible for each individual derive from the way his innate potential has been channeled in its expression by the socially determined identity he assumes. His style of mental functions, his ego structure, can be examined in group psychotherapy and the social pressure of the group can serve to reshape existing socially determined, (often family determined) patterns of social interaction and offer new ways of managing inner forces and interpersonal relationships. The ego enrichments occurring in group psychotherapy have an integrative and harmonizing effect on character distortions and deficiencies.

The current agreement that group psychotherapy is most useful for patients with personality disorders is consistent with this theoretical construct. This approach was presented at a panel discussion at the annual meeting of the American Psychiatric Association in 1965 (see Introduction).

---

* Freud, S.: *Group Psychology and the Analysis of the Ego.* London, Hogarth Press, 1948.

† Fenichel, O.: *The Psychoanalytic Theory of Neurosis.* New York, Norton, 1945, p. 464 et seq.

Through panel discussions at the annual meetings of the American Psychiatric Association and many seminars, publications, and other professional communications, group psychotherapy has continued to develop as a useful treatment technique for a broad range of patients.

Chapter 2

THE TRAINING OF THE GROUP PSYCHOTHERAPIST

The prospective group psychotherapist should be a physician who has begun his residency training in psychiatry and has had sufficient psychiatric training to recognize the diagnostic entities occurring among psychiatric patients. This book should be useful to others, however, whose training has not been along medical lines. The prospective group psychotherapist should be able to recognize the mental mechanisms patients use when they speak to him and their significance to each patient's relations with other people.

The prospective group psychotherapist should be interested in getting along with people in groups as well as individually. There are some psychiatrists whose temperament makes it impossible for them to do group psychotherapy. Group psychotherapy should not be required of them, any more than it should be required for all patients.

If the prospective group psychotherapist has had some meaningful personal psychoanalysis, this experience can prove helpful in his own self-inspection as he works with patients in groups. This is extremely valuable in learning to recognize transference reactions and to use them in treatment.

The essentials of training in group psychotherapy are as follows:

1. Supervisory sessions with a knowledgeable, flexible supervisor. These supervisory sessions can be conducted in groups or individually, but preferably in a group.

2. Sitting in an established psychotherapy group as an observer. Supervision and observation are the two most important kinds of training in group psychotherapy. Other kinds of training for the presumptive group psychotherapist include didactic

lectures, assigned reading, and at times, a group psychotherapy experience.

Because of the many problems of attempting treatment with persons who are in regular contact with one another and with the therapist outside the treatment situation, group psychotherapy experience for group psychotherapists in training involves the risk of a detrimental influence on the trainee.

Psychiatrists who are not willing to be trained in group psychotherapy should not be forced to undergo this training during the course of their residency or other training programs. Similarly, not all physicians who are interested in doing group psychotherapy are able to become practitioners of it. It should not be a reflection on the competence or integrity of any person if he is unable or unwilling to do group psychotherapy, any more than it should be a requirement of every surgeon that he do every conceivable surgical procedure.

A training program for group psychotherapists should be a part of a psychiatric residency program. In the first year of residency, the trainee may sit as an observer in an established group with a therapist, perhaps a second-year or third-year resident, who has had some training. The observer then should sit with the therapist in his supervisory sessions. The psychotherapy group should meet at least once a week for an hour and a half and should consist of from four to twelve patients. The first-year resident should be required to become familiar with two or three standard texts on group psychotherapy.

Alexander Wolf's papers in the *American Journal of Psychotherapy* should be required reading.* The book by Freeman *et al.*† should be available. The works of Eric Berne, S. H. Foulkes, J. W. Klapman, S. R. Slavson, Hugh Mullin, and Max Rosenbaum should be recommended for collateral reading.

Throughout the group psychotherapy training program its members should meet regularly to discuss the literature on group therapy and the phenomena of the groups they observe and treat.

---

* Wolf, Alexander, *loc. cit.*

† Freeman, T., Cameron, J. L., and McGhie, A.: *Chronic Schizophrenia.* New York, Int. Univs., 1958.

The discussion group should meet every week for a period ranging from sixty to ninety minutes.

During the second year of residency training, residents who wish to do so should take on a previously functioning psychotherapy group, preferably one in which the first year's observation had been done, and carry out the treatment of this group under supervision. This should be done with a first-year resident as observer, who would also attend the supervisory sessions.

During the third year, the resident should have the opportunity to organize a psychotherapy group of patients of his own selection, to which a first-year or second-year resident may be assigned.

The supervision for all three groups can be done as a group, but at least one supervisory session per week of at least one hour should be available for each therapist, if there is individual supervision. Two hours for supervision should be available if more than one therapist is to be supervised.

In the supervisory sessions, there should be a constant appraisal of the group psychotherapist's function in the group and of the functioning of the patients.

Some years ago, at a university-affiliated psychiatric residency training program, the first-year residents participated in large group sessions conducted in wards by faculty members in the group psychotherapy program. These large groups included all the patients on the ward who were able to sit still long enough to participate in a group discussion. These large groups did not represent therapy groups as such, but introduced the first-year resident to techniques in conducting groups and to the phenomena that occur in a relatively unstructured yet organized group meeting.

At appropriate times, the resident observers conducted these groups also. Immediately following these meetings, which lasted an hour, the residents discussed the phenomena observed with the supervisor, both when he conducted the group and when the resident conducted it.

The recommended reading was taken up in terms of the actual situations that occurred in the group. A few formal lectures and seminars were scheduled. Most of the teaching was done with the residents during their supervisory sessions.

During the latter part of the second year of the residency training program, the resident sat as an observer in a group conducted by one of the third-year residents. Beginning about the first of May, the second-year resident sat quietly in the group with the therapist and participated in the supervisory sessions. Around the first of July, when the resident started his third year, he took over the group in which he sat as an observer. He was supervised in his treatment of the group by the same or a different supervisor. Through his third year of residency, he continued the treatment of this group, adding and discharging patients with the help of his supervisor. During the latter part of his year with the group, he in turn received a second-year resident as an observer and prospective therapist for the group.

During this period, the resident learned many things about psychiatric diagnosis and the management of psychiatric patients. Many of these concepts were useful in working with groups. They were applied as they appeared useful and were discussed with the supervisor.

During this teaching program, questions arose of general interest to residents in training. Since they are illustrative of the problems and solutions occurring in group psychotherapy training a few of them will be discussed.

One day in this training program, after one of the large ward group meetings, Dr. L. wanted to know why the therapist had asked a mute catatonic patient what he thought about what had just been said by two other patients who had discussed their feelings of being unjustly incarcerated at this receiving hospital. The instructor who had conducted the group explained to Dr. L. that it was his practice to call on every patient at least once during each group session to give each patient an opportunity to speak. Not only the mute catatonic patient but each patient in the group was invited to speak.

This was not done all at one time as a roll call might be done, but at intervals during the group session. When a break occurred in a particular discussion or when the physician conducting the group felt it was important to terminate a discussion, he intervened in this way. In this way, each patient was drawn into the group. His comments, whether relevant to the immediately preceding comment or not, were accepted.

Gradually, in subsequent sessions, the mute catatonic patient became more responsive. Shortly before his transfer to a state hospital, he began to speak a sentence or two at each of the large group sessions. Sometimes his comments were only tangentially relevant. A clang association, sibilant response occurred at other times. However, this mute catatonic patient was drawn into the group interaction and participated in these large group sessions.

Perhaps the most important function of the supervisor in training a group psychotherapist is to support and maintain the morale of the therapist in training. The resident who first starts treating a group inevitably feels apprehensive and out of place. Until he acquires some sophistication, it is important for the supervisor to point out to him the positive aspects of what he is doing and to tell him, by giving specific examples, exactly what might be done in certain situations.

At the beginning, it is vitally important to point out to the therapist in training the constructive moves he makes without being much aware of them in his dealing with the group. It is important to show, by what he reports, how his training in psychiatry has automatically evidenced itself in his management of the therapy.

The beginning therapist may manifest his insecurity by skepticism concerning the efficacy of the treatment. He should be shown time after time how the incidents he reports of his contacts with the group illustrate the workings of the group and his own therapeutic activity.

To illustrate the way in which the supervisor may help the trainee in learning to work with the group as a modality of the treatment, the following example is given:

A resident had been treating a group of outpatients for nine months. He saw the group for one and one-half hours each week, and attended a supervisory session one hour each week with another second-year resident who was also treating a group.

At one supervisory session, he presented the problem of Mrs. S., who wanted a note or some kind of certificate from him to take to her dentist to get some discolored front teeth capped.

Mrs. S, an impulsive hysteric, had been a spinster until age twenty-nine, when a psychopathic, leather-jacketed motorcyclist met, wooed, married, impregnated, and left her, all within three months.

Mrs. S came to treatment during the latter part of this pregnancy. At the beginning, her treatment was primarily supportive and reassuring. A deliberate effort had been made to avoid raising issues that might provoke anxiety until after her child had been born and she was once again in a fairly stable situation. She lived with her mother who provided for her and did not seem too much disturbed by her adventures.

Mrs. S had continued to hear from her husband. Allegedly, he had left her to take up with a policewoman, who eventually shot him in the foot. While living with her, he had walked around the neighborhood wearing military clothing, passing himself off as one of the Green Berets.

The resident was troubled by Mrs. S's request. During his general medical training, he had been in contact with and favorably impressed by a plastic surgeon who specialized in rhinoplasty. The surgeon had explained that he had almost foolproof criteria for determining the realistic need for reconstructive operations on the nose. By using these criteria, he was supposedly able to eliminate patients who were emotionally disturbed and in need of psychiatric treatment rather than plastic surgery.

It turned out that his only criterion was that a patient who had always thought that his nose was misshapened and a hindrance to him was a case for a plastic surgeon, and that a patient who recently had decided that his nose was misshapened and a hindrance to his success was a case for a psychiatrist.

The resident considered that Mrs. S's discolored teeth could be thought of as being the same as a lifelong concern about a misshapened nose and felt inclined to do what he could to help her get the dental work that she proposed.

In the supervisory session, it was pointed out that the plastic surgeon's criterion was unrealistic and that Mrs. S represented an impulsive personality as manifested, for example, by her previous behavior in the hasty marriage. The resident was advised to help her to delay her action both as a means of teaching her to wait between feeling the urge to do something and carrying it out, and to stimulate group interaction. His previous training had taught him how to refuse to grant a patient's request without disrupting the treatment relationship.

Perhaps the most important point in this supervisory session was the emphasis on getting the resident to learn to use the group as a means of treatment. Group involvement in this problem would be likely to delay action and contribute a variety of approaches to the problem from which the patient could choose a solution, perhaps the solution of leaving her teeth alone.

It is unlikely that the other members of the group would be seduced by the patient into agreeing with her and going along with her impulsive behavior as her husband apparently had before their separation. She had also apparently persuaded her mother to be her accomplice in impulsive behavior.

At a subsequent group session, Mrs. S again presented her request for a certificate from the therapist to enable her to get her front teeth capped. The therapist declined to grant her request and referred the question to the group for discussion as the supervisor had recommended. Somewhat to the surprise of the therapist, the other members of the group made effective comments. They specifically told Mrs. S that her teeth were not her problem. As the group continued to be active in the treatment discussion it came out that Mrs. S had had a rhinoplasty and had consulted a dermatologist to request a sandpapering of her face for acne. The dermatologist had told her that her acne was not severe enough to need this kind of treatment.

During the summer another resident had advised a divorced woman who was a borderline psychotic in his group not to remarry to a man with two children by a previous marriage because he felt she had difficulty in managing her own two children. Her description of her prospective husband indicated that he had neither the time nor the money to support her emotionally or financially on other than subsistence level. She discontinued coming to the group but returned, married, the following winter. In the spring she began complaining about the difficulties she had in the marriage.

Her husband worked long hours in a retail business. His pubescent sons were a problem to her and to her eight and nine year old daughters. She was tired and discouraged, and sought the support of the therapist and the group in getting a separation and a divorce.

The advice not to marry had been given this woman by the resident who had been treating the group without supervision the preceding summer. Vacations had interfered with supervisory sessions. When the patient reappeared and asked again for direct advice, another resident who was treating the group, on the recommendation of the supervisor, avoided giving a direct recommendation. Instead he referred the patient to the group. In the group discussion, she went into how difficult it was for her to manage her newly acquired family. She complained about how ill-advised she had been. The group listened sympathetically, and the therapist remained neutral.

At the next group session she felt much relieved and better prepared to undertake the burdens of her difficult marriage. The catharsis and support reactions from the previous group session had bolstered her morale to the point where she felt she could deal more realistically with her problems.

In another instance, Mr. M, a withdrawn, compulsive man, had spoken in a derogatory way in most of his talk in group sessions over a period of two and one-half years about almost everything the other patients had brought up. He accused them of being insincere, of lacking understanding, and of really not being interested in themselves or the things they discussed.

At the recommendation of the supervisor, this patient was dealt with in a neutral fashion and allowed to express his feelings of skepticism repeatedly. Finally, in one group session where the patients were talking about work, the resident therapist intervened saying he would like to know how each felt about his own work burden. For the first time, Mr. M spoke about his own dissatisfaction with his job and how unhappy he was at work. Having been permitted to express his negative feelings and querulousness about others, he finally felt secure enough in the group to speak about the things that bothered him. Again, requiring talk from the group resulted in a therapeutic gain.

In the teaching situation there is a change of therapist as residents pass through their training program. This change can be utilized in the teaching of the residents and treatment of the groups of patients.

Dr. A for example, had been conducting group therapy with outpatients in the teaching hospital clinic since July of the preceding year. In April he was advised to tell the group that another therapist would be coming soon, but to give no definite time for the appearance of the new therapist until he was absolutely sure of the date. When the prospective new therapist learned in May the date of his arrival, Dr. A then told the group that Dr. B would probably start treating the group in July and would be sitting with the group at their regular meetings. Dr. B had been instructed to sit quietly as an observer with the group. He had made arrangements to attend the supervisory sessions with Dr. A.

Dr. A was instructed to mention that he was leaving in July at least once in every group meeting, early enough in each session to allow time for comments by the members of the group. This was done to allow the patients to vent their feelings about the change in therapists. This, of course, related to past separations from parents, siblings, and others with whom they had been in close contact and with whom they had developed important emotional ties. This aspect of the group therapy is very essential to their working out the feeling of past losses due to separations from persons important to them.

The time of changing over from one therapist to the next is crucial for the patients as well as the trainee therapist. The supervisor must be ready for tension-provoking incidents to occur with the therapists in training during this period.

Chapter 3

THE SELECTION AND PREPARATION
OF PATIENTS

Patients to be selected for group psychotherapy should first be seen in individual psychiatric consultation. At the time the consultation is made, the kinds of treatment considered feasible for the patient should be noted. When the patient is seen first by a consultant other than the prospective group psychotherapist, the group therapist must decide later, on the basis of his own contact with the patient, whether he feels he can work with this patient in a group.

At times it is necessary to have several interviews with a patient before he can be properly evaluated for group therapy. At other times, patients will be placed in group therapy on a trial basis.

An important factor in the success or failure of a patient's participation in group psychotherapy is the attitude of the therapist. Group psychotherapy has its indications that are as positive and definite as the indications for any other kind of medical treatment. Flexibility in patient management is much easier for a therapist who clearly understands the risks of the course of action that he takes in the management of a patient. The fact that group psychotherapy is indicated and carried out in a given case does not preclude individual visits, use of medication, somatic treatments, hospitalization, or any of the other available treatment modalities.

Generally, the patients suitable for group psychotherapy are those who are severely neurotic, borderline cases, and remitted psychotics who have some tolerance for the psychotherapy. The combination of supportive and integrative therapy available to each patient in a group lends itself to the treatment of these cases.* This comprises the bulk of patients applying for treatment. While probably not suitable for most treatment services, outpatient psychiatric services have been conducted in which group psychotherapy was the primary psychotherapeutic modality. Patients with acute psychotic reactions can be treated in group psychotherapy; in these cases, however, the technique must be modified to lend itself to the place of treatment. The symptom neurotics are most suitable for psychoanalysis or individual integrative psychotherapy as the treatment of choice because of their transference reactions. Severely depressed patients should be treated with drugs and other techniques, but may be helped by group treatment after the depressive episode has remitted.[1]

One general indication for group psychotherapy is the inability of the patient to communicate well enough to participate in individual psychotherapy. Patients whose styles of communication are overproductive or underproductive, or characterized by activity rather than words often do better in groups than in attempts at individual treatment. It should be understood that group psychotherapy does not preclude individual psychotherapy in these cases. Group psychotherapy is an extremely flexible form of treatment that can be combined with many other kinds of psychiatric treatment.

The patient who does not speak in a group can listen. Often, such a patient will sit quietly for several sessions before speaking. Ultimately, he will break his silence as he becomes more interested in the talk and the group pressure to participate increases.

The patient who is overtalkative has to be restrained at times by the therapist and at other times by the group; the latter is preferable. The other patients in the group should tell him when he talks so much that he interferes with the opportunities of the other patients to speak.

Patients who are inclined to act rather than communicate, who often do things without thinking and then regret the consequences, are inclined to sit quietly and often impatiently in the group. Their first verbal communications are usually not responsive to

---

* Pinney, E. L., Jr.: "The Psychiatric Indications for Group Psychotherapy." *loc. cit.*

[1] The One Hundred and Twenty-first Annual Meeting of the American Psychiatric Association, 1965. *op. cit.*

preceding talk in the group, and these patients are inclined not to wait for answers to their questions but to go on talking about their own interests. Eventually, this is pointed out to them by the group or the therapist. These patients learn first, however, to communicate and then how to evaluate and respond to the content of communications.

The communicative aspect of group psychotherapy works out in the composition of the group. The group must have in common enough social and economic background for meaningful communication and interactions to occur. Although not all members of a psychotherapy group need to have the same socioeconomic status, there has to be a common knowledge of the attitudes and styles of socioeconomic practice among the group members. In the selection of patients for a particular group, its socioeconomic composition ordinarily takes precedence over the diagnostic categories. Although psychotherapy groups assembled on the basis of diagnostic category alone can be helpful to the patients, the degree of functional impairment and the socioeconomic factors have a relatively greater influence in the composition of a working psychotherapy group.

Another kind of patient who can benefit from group psychotherapy enormously is the one who communicates fairly well verbally but whose thinking is unusual; for instance, the patient who almost never speaks to the point and never gets to the main issue. Gradually in the course of group discussion, this aspect of his talk becomes obvious and the impact of the group as they repeatedly question and correct him gives the the patient an opportunity to be aware of the reaction of others to what he does. This may help him to be more flexible and less rigid, at the least; at best, he may learn to evaluate his thinking in terms of his experiences in the group.

An example of this kind of patient is Mrs. N, a chronic paranoid schizophrenic woman with two small children. She was inclined to take seriously almost every rule of child raising that she came across. Luckily for her, the group discussion led her to question precepts that she felt at first inclined to apply rigidly. Her inherent schizophrenic doubt was utilized to provide a flexibility in her relationships with her children. The group treatment helped relieve her anxiety. Her way of management enabled her children to function adequately with their playmates in a regular school setting.

The relationship of the patient to the therapist makes individual and group psychotherapy possible. The group psychotherapist should have a good understanding of himself and a good understanding of psychopathology and psychodynamics in order to recognize the important elements of the relationships that occur with each patient and within psychotherapy groups. Ordinarily, patients who are going to be treated in group psychotherapy have been seen individually several times for evaluation and for treatment before being admitted to a group. At times it will be important to continue individual sessions for a patient during the course of his group psychotherapy. When group psychotherapy is the primary treatment for a patient, individual interviews may be necessary from time to time.

When group psychotherapy is recommended to a patient, the recommendation should be made in the same style as any other recommendation for treatment. The patient is told directly that it is the doctor's opinion that the best kind of treatment for his kind of trouble is group psychotherapy. The therapist may explain to the patient that other kinds of treatment will be available to him when they appear to be in his best interest. This recommendation is made within the framework of the doctor-patient relationship in the same manner as any other recommendation for a treatment that is expected to be expensive, at times difficult, for the patient and expected to result in meaningful change in his functioning. When group pyschotherapy is properly recommended, the patient will submit to this treatment in the same way as patients submit to medical treatment recommended for other conditions.

Owing to the popular belief that all psychotherapy requires the patient to speak whatever comes into his mind, the patient often believes that he may expose himself completely when talking at a group session. Patients must be told that in group psychotherapy, as opposed to psychoanalysis and some kinds of psychoanalytic treatment, they are not required to free associate but only to say what appears appropriate at the time. That what they feel impelled to speak about or to omit may be questioned in the group may be called to their attention also. It is not necessary for each patient to speak his thoughts as in free association. From the practical standpoint, this is impossible in a group anyhow. The areas of reactive overemphasis and phobic omission will make themselves evident eventually in the group conversations of the treatment.

A twenty-year-old white woman, Mrs. E, had come for private consultation two weeks before her marriage. Her complaint was that she feared crowds and traveling. This trouble had begun during the courtship with her prospective husband. It had led to her becoming increasingly anxious and disabled. She had been working as an executive secretary in a nationally known company. She had finally given up her job because overwhelming anxiety had made her so uncomfortable.

She described her mother as a very fearful woman who almost never left home. A maternal uncle was a chronic patient in a state hospital. Mrs. E herself had never had friendly relations with her peers, although she had been active in extracurricular activities at school and had done well in her studies. She had been brought up to observe her religious faith strictly.

The physician's talking to her and her prospective husband at the end of the consultation failed to persuade them to postpone the marriage. She seemed amenable to psychotherapy. However, the extreme degree of disability and the almost complete pervasion of all areas of function by symptoms, plus a lack of dimensions of movement in the history of her past adjustment, indicated that group psychotherapy would be helpful to her. Accordingly, she was told that her treatment would include medication to relieve her tension, individual psychotherapy, and perhaps at a future date group psychotherapy. This course of treatment was followed.

Mrs. E was seen for nineteen months in individual psychotherapy during which time she made some symptomatic improvement. She had gotten married and as was to be expected, had begun to have difficulty with her husband. Although she was able to function as a housewife, she continued to be handicapped by being unable to shop or attend religious services regularly.

She and her husband decided that she should become pregnant. It seemed useless to try to dissuade them just as it had been useless to try to get them to postpone the marriage. The patient discontinued treatment for five months, from her eighth month of pregnancy until her son was four months old.

Mrs. E had become a little more aware of the emotional factors in her daily living. She had begun to examine some of the influences of her parents and siblings on her personality development. She continued to be afraid the therapist might be missing a brain tumor or might otherwise do or omit something that might result in a physical medical disaster for her and her child or that he would lead her to commit some immoral behavior that would endanger her immortal soul. She had, however, developed enough confidence in the therapist and enough awareness of the nonassaultive attitudes of people generally that she was willing to begin group psychotherapy.

She then returned to treatment and at this time agreed to the replacement of one of her individual psychotherapy sessions by one group psychotherapy session a week. Individual psychotherapy was continued for eleven months after the patient had started group therapy. At that point, the individual appointments were made optional. At times they were recommended by the therapist and at other times arranged at the request of the patient.

Mr. M, a twenty-year-old college student, complained of difficulty in sleeping and in concentrating and studying. When he was eight years old, his father, a promising engineer, had died of leukemia. His mother had remarried when he was fifteen. The stepfather had been a boorish alcoholic who had had to give up his drinking when he developed mild diabetes. Mr. M had not done well in high school. He had received barely passing grades, although psychological testing at the time of consultation had shown that he was of superior intelligence. Three months prior to the psychiatric consultation, he had taken LSD "trips." His present complaints had begun a month subsequent to the second dose of LSD.

At interview, he presented himself as a lonely, socially isolated, mildly depressed young man who wanted help with problems he felt to be very painful. He was oriented and in good contact with his environment. He spent much of his time alone, sometimes playing his guitar. He affected a clean and orderly but informal style of dress, bordering on that of a beatnik. He reported having seen "an orange square" one evening as he sat in his room staring at the wall.

He was immediately started in individual psychotherapy with one session a week of group psychotherapy. His poor social relationships and isolation indicated unfulfilled personality needs that he could fulfill with devices provided by group psychotherapy. The organic signs probably related to LSD ingestion. The irritability leading to insomnia and the visual hallucination indicated the need for supportive management. This function the group provided in addition to the supportive aspect of the individual psychotherapy.

By contrast, Mr. T, a twenty-seven-year-old stockbroker trainee, came for psychiatric consultation complaining of "dizzy spells" that turned out to be anxiety states related to traveling by train to his job and to walking on the street with fellow employees. Mr. T was married and the father of a two-year-old son. He had recently purchased his own home and had been promised a seat on the New York Stock Exchange by his firm within a relatively short time. His social relationships were satisfactory. His family history was notable in that he had far surpassed his father financially and occupationally, the father having been a freight elevator operator all his life.

The precipitating factor in Mr. T's symptoms was a telephone call suggesting a sexual affair that he received at home one evening from a woman who frequented the bowling alley where Mr. T went regularly with friends. At the time he received the call his wife and child were away from home. The immediate aim in treatment was to get the patient stabilized at his present functional level.

Mr. T's diagnosis was anxiety reaction. His overt transference reaction was a positive, hopeful feeling toward the therapist, tinged with fear that some terrible physical catastrophe would occur, leaving him crippled or dead. His hostile feelings could be handled better in the intimacy of a one-to-one treatment than in a group where they could not be easily presented.

The support of the group was not required by this patient in his direct encounters with the therapist. Neither did he need the feeling that the presence of the other patients would prevent him from committing some atrocity.

Mr. T was treated with individual psychotherapy twice a week and showed significant improvement after eighteen months of treatment. He did not have the personality pattern nor trait difficulties that would have made him most likely to need the contributions group psychotherapy could offer to his feeling of identity or his personality organization.

Chapter 4

THE CHARACTER OF THE GROUP

Groups in which a certain number of patients are selected for group psychotherapy and no new patients are added during its course, which is for a limited period, are called closed groups. Closed groups are useful for study and teaching, but not suitable for carrying on long-range treatment.

Most patients need care in a setting that can be extended over long periods of time. Patients sometimes will be able to get along without treatment for long intervals and then must resume it. A closed group precludes this possibility. Some patients improve more rapidly than others and have no need to continue treatment further at that point. To continue to carry them because an arbitrary length of time has been set for the life of the group is unrealistic.

Open psychotherapy groups are those in which new patients enter and old patients drop out from time to time. Open groups begin when a group psychotherapist gets enough patients together to start one and continue indefinitely. New patients are added as old patients leave. Open groups allow patients to enter group psychotherapy, stay for a while, leave, and return as needed.

The goals of treatment can be reached and modified according to the needs and abilities of the patients as the group continues. Defining the goals of treatment in terms of assisting patients to perform better and more comfortably in their day-to-day living can be carried out most easily in an open group.

The character of the group is determined by the setting and the therapist. Captive groups are those made up of patients in hospitals, other institutions, prisons, and outpatients who are placed in groups during the time they are required to see a psychiatrist by a court or during the aftercare or convalescent status required following hospitalization in a public hospital.

Free groups are made up of patients who voluntarily come for treatment to a clinic, doctor's office, or other setting in which the patient voluntarily submits to group treatment and voluntarily continues it. It is possible for a free group to function within a hospital or other setting in which patients are incarcerated; however, the usual practice for patients who are confined is that they are already confined to the area in which the group meets or that they be brought to it.

The therapist decides the kind of patients he can and is willing and able to work with. He selects his patients on that basis. Doctors who work in state hospitals would be expected to work most of the time with captive groups of psychotic patients. Prison psychiatrists might also work with captive groups of psychotics, but one would expect them to see more patients with personality disorders.

In institutional settings, patients are likely to be all of the same sex in the therapy group because patients are ordinarily segregated on this basis. However, mixed male and female groups do occur in such settings. The opportunity for mixed male and female groups occurs more frequently in free groups in outpatient settings.

Groups in which patients are all of the same sex and all of the same general diagnostic category may be thought of as homogeneous. Even in these groups there are many differences between patients which give rise to therapeutic interaction. Most groups, however, are heterogeneous in diagnostic, age, and occupational makeup, if not of mixed gender.

An obvious selection goes on of patients to bring into and to remain in therapeutic groups which is the result of the therapist's personality. Some therapists are only comfortable with a group of docile, well-behaved patients with whom the talk may appear to be only polite chitchat. At the other extreme, there are therapists who somehow manage to have loud, raucous group sessions at every meeting.

The therapist should be aware of his preferences and consider them in his selection of patients. At times, he should take patients on the basis of suitability for treatment who are not the type he finds it most gratifying to work with. In meaningful psychotherapy, the therapist must deprive himself as well as the patient.

This is an important distinction between therapeutic relationships and ordinary social relationships.

In the selection of patients for a group in private practice, variations in cultural and educational background can be tolerated easily, provided the general aims and motivations of the patients in the group have some similarities. For instance, one group of women who had in common their having worked in an office, mostly as stenographers, functioned very well. Their business and occupational interests served to highlight their mutual problems in marriage and courtship or as a spinster career woman.

In this group, the educational level varied from high school to postgraduate college. The economic status varied also, from bare subsistence to affluence. The problems of these women concerning femininity and identity had a common language and common orientation.

Another group of women consisted of patients who had been somewhat more disorganized. Most of them were single. They had never settled down to regular employment, with the exception of one or two severely obsessive-compulsive patients who had stayed at the same job for years. They doubted everything. In a sense, the consistent questioning of these patients was a constant element. Again, the group setting provided a kind of heterogeneous identity committee to help them and the other members of the group sort out and decide which better courses to follow in running their lives.

Chapter 5

THE FIRST MEETINGS OF A NEW GROUP

After a number of patients, usually more than three and less than thirteen, have been selected for a group, the group psychotherapist sets the time and place for their first meeting. At this meeting the patients are strangers to one another. Each patient has become acquainted previously with the therapist during his individual sessions. This relationship of the therapist to each patient and his authority as an expert who can help him to help himself are the grounds for the organization and functioning of the therapeutic group.

Implicit in the communications of the therapist is the message that the patients get together for treatment and for no other purpose. Group psychotherapy is not a substitute for social relationships. Each patient's problems in socialization can be helped by the treatment process in group psychotherapy, but the group psychotherapy itself is no substitute for an adequate social life. One of the deprivations that the patient and the therapist must undergo in this kind of treatment is the necessity for maintaining the discipline of the therapeutic task in the treatment, rather than allowing themselves the social gratifications possible in such a setting.

At the initial session of a group, patients are confused and need guidance from the therapist in how to go about the work of the group treatment. One way to start the group at its work is to poll the group informally by asking "What do you think we should be doing here?"

Checking with a representative number of the group members to obtain a consensus and dissents from it ordinarily assures adequate and lively group discussion at the beginning. Once this kind of interaction has begun, the work of the group is underway.

It is important that the therapist avoid the kinds of questions that might be categorized as "Guess what I am thinking." At times the therapist should directly intervene with a clear statement. Almost all of the time the consensus of the group with its dissents will provide a close enough approximation to the general reality that no emendation from the therapist is required.

At the first group meeting, the group psychotherapist can expect to do most of the talking. He persuades, explains, and questions. His duty is to teach the patients that they can work together. His explanations are more effective if they are related to examples drawn from the group interaction. The here-and-now examples that he can give will have a pungency that analogy and stories about other groups and other situations cannot possibly have.

Dr. Y had been trained during his residency to do group psychotherapy. As a part of his training he had treated both inpatient and outpatient groups under supervision. His orientation had been psychoanalytic and his expectation in private practice had been to do individual integrative psychotherapy.

In his first months of practice, several of the patients who had been referred to him did not do well in individual treatment. Most had severe personality disorders, a few were remitted psychotics, and some were chronic schizophrenics.

The transference reactions of these patients were marked by fearfulness, suspicion, antagonism, and irritability, along with more positive feelings and the desire for some help. Countertransference reactions of irritation, boredom, and somnolence were a problem.

Finally, Dr. Y decided that he could put to good use the techniques he had learned in his training by gathering these patients together and treating them in a group.

After telling the patients that he felt group psychotherapy would be useful to them and discussing his proposal a few times in the individual sessions, Dr. Y found that most of these patients were willing to undergo this kind of treatment. The patients had their doubts, of course, but their doubts represented the same kinds of skepticism related to individual psychotherapy.

Two patients discontinued treatment during the time Dr. Y was discussing the possibility of group psychotherapy with them. These patients had not consistently kept their appointments, nor had they been reliable enough to be more than only fair candidates for any kind of psychotherapy.

When the patients got together for the first group meeting, they had in common their acquaintance with Dr. Y. They were familiar with him and his style of working. However, they learned at the first session that his approach and behavior as a group psychotherapist differed from his technique in individual sessions. Some patients had expected in the group the same kind of one-to-one relationship with the therapist that had taken place in the individual sessions. They were dismayed to find, for instance, that questions from them to the therapist were deflected to other members of the group.

At this first meeting Dr. Y began the session by asking, "What do you think we should do here?"

One of the more anxious and ingratiating patients immediately began a sycophant-like recital of his version of group psychotherapy as derived from seeing motion pictures and television programs and from reading popular literature. He omitted what had been told him about group psychotherapy during the individual sessions. The other patients who had been told that it was a kind of treatment that was likely to help them with their problems and that the other patients in the group were people who would have somewhat similar problems reacted immediately to what had been said. The talk of the group psychotherapy had begun and the first meeting of this group moved into an active discussion. The therapeutic work had begun. Within fifteen minutes, the therapist's work had became guiding rather than initiating the discussion.

The transference dilution in the group makes it easy for the negative feelings of each individual patient to be dissipated among several objects. The troublesome countertransferences were thereby not so strongly evoked. The behavior of the patients in the group, based on these transference reactions, can be recognized by the therapist and other members in the group for the inappropriate emotions that they are and can be handled much more readily in the group treatment setting than in individual psychotherapy.

At a public hospital clinic, a number of severely ill patients had been organized into a group because they were felt to be refractory to individual psychotherapy and not cooperative enough to follow through consistently with drug treatment and other treatment modalities offered them.

At the first group meeting, many negative feelings were expressed. The general tone was antiauthoritarian, directed against people in the guardian or helping positions for these adults. These patients viewed the group as just another way of being brushed off and ignored. Several of them did not return for follow-up. However, the opportunity to speak and listen to others with similar complaints intrigued most of the patients. They attended subsequent sessions regularly.

The position of the therapist with this group was one of an indulgent parent who listened to the complaints of his angry children, recognizing as they did among themselves that the complaints were irrational, yet helping them to express and thereby relieve themselves enough of the anger to permit some worthwhile advances.

The first meeting of the group was characterized by the variety of patient responses. A few were entirely inappropriate for group psychotherapy. Most of the patients who were consistently inappropriate eliminated themselves from the group by not returning.

In more than one case, however, this one group meeting had the effect of encouraging the patients to attend more carefully the drug treatment routines that had been set up for them. Some of the patients took support from the presence of the others and spoke freely to a psychiatrist for the first time. This, for them, was the beginning of some meaningful treatment. This group of severely ill outpatients resembled the large group of patients in a hospital ward meeting conducted for training purposes.

There were eleven adults, both men and women, for this first group session. Most of them were severely and chronically mentally ill, although only a few had been psychiatrically hospitalized. Patients were called from the waiting room and brought to a conference room, where they sat in chairs placed around a large table. The therapist began by introducing himself, saying, "I am Dr. ——"; then, going completely around the group, he asked each patient in turn, "What is your name?"

Some verbatim extracts of this group session follow:

THE FIRST MEETING OF A NEW GROUP

DOCTOR: I'm Dr. ——. What is your name? M. C.?

M. C.: Yes.

DOCTOR: And Mr. V? And your name?

ANSWER: Nora C.

DOCTOR: And you're Mr. E?

MR. E.: No, Joe E.

DOCTOR: And your name?

ANSWER: A. D.

DOCTOR: And your name?

ANSWER: Miss I.

DOCTOR: And you?

ANSWER: Mr. N.

(And so on)

* * *

DOCTOR: Do you have any idea what we should be doing here?

MISS Q: We've got our problems.

DOCTOR: What do you think we do here?

MR. D: I'm here because I have an appointment for today.

DOCTER: Mr. V, do you know what we are supposed to do here? And you, Mr. E? Have you ever been in anything like this before?

MR. E: No.

* * *

DOCTOR: Miss N, do you have any idea what this is all about?

MISS N: Well, I don't know if this is like it used to be, but we used to talk and solve each other's problems. (This patient had participated in an activity group at another clinic.)

DOCTOR: And your name?

ANSWER: Miss T.

DOCTOR: How do you spell it?

MISS T: (Spells her name)

DOCTOR: And your first name?

MISS T: (Says her first name)

DOCTOR: Miss I, do you have any idea what we do here?

MISS I: No, I don't. It's the first time I've been to something like this.

DOCTOR: Miss T, do you know anything about this, what we do here? Mr. N, what do you think?

MR. N: Asking questions, how are you, why you're depressed, why you're so and so, when you're going to take things in your own hands, that's what it is.

DOCTOR: Do you agree with him, Miss Q?

MISS Q: Yes.

DOCTOR: Mrs. D, do you understand any of this? Let her tell me, if she will.

* * *

DOCTOR: Now, we meet here ordinarily at ten-thirty Friday mornings and we'll talk until some time around noon. (The therapist presents the schedule of meetings.)

MRS. I: Excuse me, I can't very well do that because I have children that go to school and they have to leave school at twelve-thirty.

DOCTOR: Well, make whatever arrangements you can. It's up to you.

MR. N: How about one o'clock?

MISS Q: No, I have to go to work.

DOCTOR: Maybe you can make some arrangement to have someone help you with the children.

MRS. I: I haven't anybody to help me, my husband works.

DOCTOR: What do you think about it, Mr. E?

MR. E: It's her problem.

DOCTOR: Miss D, what do you think?

MISS D: I'm just listening.

DOCTOR: Do you find it interesting?

MISS D: Yes.

DOCTOR: What is it for? What do you think it's for, Mr. V?

MR. V: I'm just listening also.

DOCTOR: Miss Q?

MISS T: Why do you need a tape recorder?

DOCTOR: So that I have a record of what happens.

MISS Q: Don't you have to have our consent before you can take it?

DOCTOR: It's here.

MISS Q: I found that out with Dr. ——.

DOCTOR: If you don't want to be taped, you may leave. This is consent; it's here.

MISS Q: Okay.

DOCTOR: There is nothing hidden about it, you see. You want to know what you are here for? (This takes up the question raised previously. The purpose of this intervention is to focus the attention of the patients on the work of the group.)

MR. E: Yes.

DOCTOR: That's a good question. What are you here for, Mr. D?

MR. D: To keep the appointment that I have or what would I be here for?

MISS T: Don't you know?

DOCTOR: Do you know why he's here?

MISS T: That same reason everyone else is here.

DOCTOR: What's that? Did you come here for help, Mr. E?

MR. E: I was sent down here from upstairs, and they was trying to find out my problem. I talked with the social worker the other day, the early part of this week, and I still don't understand nothing. They didn't say there was something wrong with me, whether there was or nothing.

DOCTOR: You think you might be here in good health then? (Quietly and soberly).

MR. E: I don't know, nobody has told me nothing. All they did was I was examined and they never told me nothing. I figure a guy should know what's wrong with him.

DOCTOR: What do you think about that, Miss Q?

MISS Q: I think that too.

DOCTOR: How do you account for the fact that he comes here all this time and doesn't know what is wrong with him? (This intervention was designed to call attention to the denial of illness expressed in Mr. E's previous statement.)

Miss Q: You had a complaint and they couldn't find anything wrong with you?

Mr. E: Well, you know a physical defect on my right side, but they was talking to me about drinking, you know?

Miss Q: Oh.

Doctor: Do you drink too much?

Mr. E: Yes, I drink an excess amount, yes.

Doctor: Well, maybe that has something to do with what is wrong with you.

Mr. E: I thought this was a psychiatric treatment, you know?

Doctor: Do you think this is a psychiatric treatment, Miss N?

Miss N: Well, I think yes, in a way, in other words, just like I said before, we're going to try to help iron out the problems we have. Some people may have different problems. I may have affairs, maybe drink, maybe somebody might do this, now this helps us iron out our problems.

Doctor: How does that sound to you, Mr. D? Did you hear what she said? Can you tell him again, Miss N?

Miss N: Some people may have affairs. Maybe some people may have alcoholic problems, some may have dope problems—you don't know—maybe they try to see if they can get away from these problems.

Doctor: You understand?

Mr. D: Yes.

Doctor: Miss T, what do you think about it?

Miss T: I don't drink, and—

Doctor: Are you here for trouble of some kind?

Miss T: Yes.

Doctor: What kind of trouble are you here for, can you tell us?

Miss T: Problems. (Here is the answer. Miss T has told Mr. E that she is here for "problems.")

Mr. N: Doctor, why don't we have like a dance instead of asking questions, and make everyone happy? (Another attempt at denial and to evade treatment by saying it is not the kind of thing he had in mind as "treatment.")

Doctor: What about that, do you want to have a dance?

Mr. N: Yes, that's a good idea. (The attempt at denial of

emotional difficulty and of the fact the group represents psychiatric treatment immediately recurs.)

Mr. E: What's the use of dancing and having fun to make somebody forget their troubles? Like when I drink, when I finish drinking, I wake up sober—I still have the same problems then. That doesn't solve anything.

Miss N: That's right.

Doctor: Mrs. I, what do you think about it?

Mrs. I: Well, I don't know, I'm just here. But I don't even know what I'm here for. I received a letter to come in today, and I wasn't supposed to come here until the twenty-second. I didn't know what it was all about. I thought they were bringing me here today to ask questions with a doctor.

Doctor: Well, I'm a doctor, you know. (The therapist calls attention to himself as a doctor, which again reiterates his function in treating illness. If he agreed to having a dance, he would then be a dancing master and go along with the denial of illness. This is not to be construed that recreational activities are not worthwhile for patients. They are; however, they are distinct from the specific treatment.)

Mrs. I: No, with the other doctor, you know, personally— just the doctor and yourself. Like I was here before and they told me I was supposed to come back the twenty-second and they sent me a letter and I had to take my children out of school in order to come here.

Doctor: It seems that you've gone to a great deal of trouble to get here.

Mrs. I: Yes, I have.

Doctor: You're really concerned about this?

Mrs. I: Of course I am. I don't know what's going on, what's happening.

Doctor: Well, it's a good question, what's going on and what's happening? (Turning the questions to the group.)

Mr. N: Doctor, how come a guy like me always gets a place, stays in the house, and nobody wants to talk to him, and everybody moves away from him? I'm all alone. (This patient takes up the problems he has and the group begins to talk about their problems.)

DOCTOR: Anything like that happen to you, Mr. D?

MR. N: It happened to me.

DOCTOR: Does it happen to you?

MISS Q: People don't stay away from me, I stay away from people.

DOCTOR: You stay away from people.

MR. N: Can I ask you one question? My people got old houses, you see. And they don't want to do nothing with me, only in case you get sick, they want to know you. Now what do they do that for? I'm their flesh and blood. I am.

DOCTOR: Let's see what Mrs. I thinks about this.

MRS. I: Well, I think he should go out and make new friends, meet people, a job, find himself some extra work to do.

MR. N: Who's going to give me a job?

DOCTOR: Wait, now let's see what you think about it. What do you think about it, Mr. E? (The therapist has taken the concern of Mr. N around to other members of the group. They have become involved and the cohesiveness of the group is apparent.)

MR. E: I think like this. If people don't want to be bothered with you, why put yourself off on people? Like, leave them alone, you know?

DOCTOR: Mr. V? Any comment? All right. Miss N?

MISS N: Well, people get tired of other people's problems, they tell you they got their own. Well, I'm thinking if they've got their own, that's what psychiatrists and doctors are for, to go to. For instance, in the last few weeks, I've been to the place where I had so much fear about everything, I haven't been able to do anything in my house. When I get in that kind of attitude and I'm afraid to walk through the street, then I need to see a doctor.

DOCTOR: Did anything like that happen to you, Mr. E?

MR. E: My case is entirely different. You see, it's like this. I don't get no spells, I don't get no fallout. I got problems, but I don't worry about them. When I drink, I drink about everything. I drink about thirty-five dollars' worth of alcohol a week.

But I don't drink it because of my problems, I just drink it with the fellows, at a party, that's all. Then I come home, I go to sleep.

Miss T: Just social?

Mr. E: It's a little more than social. You see, all the fellows in my crowd, they're big drinkers. You see, I've been drinking since I've been thirteen years old. It's become a part of me. I don't drink for a problem. I just drink to be drinking.

Doctor: What do you think would happen if you didn't drink?

Mr. E: I start hurting. I tried it once. I started hurting in my stomach.

Miss N: I don't drink. I've been smoking since I was ten.

Doctor: (To another patient) What do you do? Are you a drinker or a smoker?

Miss N: I'm a smoker too. I've been smoking so many cigarettes.

Miss T: How long have you been smoking?

Miss N: Since I was ten.

Miss T: You too?

Doctor: Mr. D, why do you think Mr. E drinks so much?

Mr. D: I don't know.

Doctor: Do you drink?

Mr. D: No.

Miss T: I think I know why he drinks.

Mr. E: Why?

Miss T: To forget sorrows.

Mr. E: I have none.

Miss Q: Then what do you come down here for?

Miss T: That's what everybody says.

Mrs. I: Now you just can't do without it, can you? You've been drinking so long?

Mr. E: That's just about the size of it. I'm going to have to drink all my life. I just take the world as it is, bad as it is.

Miss T: You and everybody else.

Mr. E: No, I wouldn't say everybody else. I make the decision myself. I don't worry where I have to turn to somebody else to solve this problem.

MISS T: But you are.

MR. E: Okay, when I was thirteen years old, did I have a problem?

DOCTOR: Why not?

MR. E: At thirteen?

DOCTOR: At thirteen.

MISS N: You can have a problem. A family problem.

MR. E: No. I came from a wealthy family, everything was pretty good, it still is. My mother and father have been married forty-five years now.

MISS N: Maybe you don't have a family problem. There are kids that get everything they want, but they still don't get enough loving.

MR. E: As a matter of fact, I was most fortunate. When I first started to drink, me and my brothers, we went south. I was about thirteen, my brothers were a little older, but we was on the farm for about two years, just to learn how to work, you know. My parents sent us down there so we wouldn't grow up like a bum, you know, to learn us how to work. So while we was down there we started drinking corn liquor and that was how it started. When I came back we was still drinking. None of us stopped. But I didn't have no problems.

(Mr. E has stopped his blatant denial and has talked about some of his problems. The therapist does not let the group reach any one conclusion. He avoids closure by taking the matter around to other patients and again encounters denial.)

DOCTOR: What do you think, Mr. V? Mr. D, did you hear what he said? Mrs. Da (who had been talking to another patient), are you through? Are you finished? What do you think we do, what do you think we're here for?

MRS. Da: I don't know.

DOCTOR: It's a good question, what this meeting is all about, what we're here for.

MISS G: I've got a pretty good idea.

MR. E: I've got an idea now too.

DOCTOR: Can you tell us about it?

MR. E: Well, when I was in school I used to go for speech

classes, you know, a lot of kids would sit around and we'd all say different sounds with our mouth, and the teacher would take this down in the record, then we'd get each kid individually and try to help that person out and see how we would react in a group; with strange people that he had never met before, how would he take to the people, how he would act or be able to adapt.

DOCTOR: Is that the way you see it? Miss T?

MISS T: I never went to speech class in all my life and I don't want to. I don't see it that way. I see it in something other than that. I'm trying to get help.

DOCTOR: Mr. D, do you think this might have something to do with helping people?

MR. D: I don't know.

DOCTOR: Mr. V, what do you think?

MR. E: I don't think it can help you too much.

DOCTOR: What were you thinking, Miss N?

MISS N: It helps people, I can say that.

MRS. Da: I don't know, you ask me that question because I was in my—I don't know what you're talking about.

(The denial is used in the discussion to keep up the work of the group.)

* * *

MISS T: I'm talking to Mr. E. I come from a wealthy family, what does it prove?

MR. E: It doesn't prove anything. I only used it to show you the point where I don't see where I have problems at home where I drink too much.

MISS N: You just picked up a habit, that's all. The same way you pick it up, you have to try to get off it. That's all.

MISS Q: What are you here for? Say something intelligent.

MR. V: Like what?

MISS Q: E equals M square, something like that. What are you here for, just to listen?

MR. V: Yes.

DOCTOR: Well, would you let him listen?

MISS Q: He can listen, but I think he should participate. Actually, the group inhibits people. It keeps them from discussing their innermost problems; you want to discuss that with the doctor.

DOCTOR: I see. Do you feel inhibited, Mr. E? (The therapist meets Miss Q's hostile destructive provocation with a bland "I see" and carried her questions and doubts to Mr. E, then to Mr. D, then to Mrs. I, and finally back to Miss Q. The irrational attack is dissipated and the inaccuracy of Miss Q's statements is shown. Miss Q's long-absent father and the sadomasochistic relation she has with her mother probably determine the transference aspect of this bit of her behavior.)

MR. E: I was sitting around here talking, and I still really don't have a full understanding of the problem.

DOCTOR: Mr. D, do you understand what he says?

MR. D: No.

DOCTOR: Mrs. I, what do you think about this?

MRS. I: Yes. Well, I agree with them because I still don't know what is going on myself.

MISS Q: Also, the group is just about the only thing we're offered down here. There is no individual therapy.

DOCTOR: Is that right?

MISS Q: Well, I don't have any.

MR. E: I have.

MISS T: I have.

MISS Q: I've had it. Actually I've had better care here than at the other hospitals. This was last year though, better care than at other hospitals, but right now, it's just the group.

(Several patients talk at once about their past experiences at clinics).

DOCTOR: Wait please—sorry. We have to do one at a time or we won't get anywhere. You've had some treatment before, Mr. E?

MR. E: Only during—let's see, I had about three. The session here and last month, the first time I've ever been down here.

MISS Q: You know, we had a very good group going before.

MR. N: That's right.

MISS Q: We did—the best group this hospital ever had—with ——.

MR. E: How did the group start? It's the first time a lot of us have been here together like this. Like when you was in the group before, when you first met each other, how did it start?

(The group interaction becomes more heated and productive.)

MISS Q: I didn't say anything because I felt strange around people. But after awhile I talked and talked and talked, but I didn't really talk about what was really bothering me because all these people around, I didn't want to tell them my problems, so I talked about symptoms and stuff.

DOCTOR: Do you think this is the way Mr. V feels?

MR. V: I didn't say that.

MISS Q: Have you ever been in group therapy before?

MISS N: Can I ask this? Is this the place where open problems should be discussed?

DOCTOR: It can be.

MISS N: I mean, I'm not ashamed of my problems. Because I want some help. About three weeks ago I had a death in my family and I went into a nervous shock and I had a doctor to come in to take care of me and he gave me narcotics that were too strong for me and it's been pulling my body down ever since I went into it, and from one thing to the other thing it's not making me feel no better and it don't seem to be taking me out of the shock, all I'm doing is shaking and the reactions from the medicines and what not, and all I'm doing is going to the doctor and spending my money and I'm not getting no better.

(The therapist rather passively carries questions from one patient to another. This involved nonparticipation is actually quite directive, although to patients it appears that the therapist is "not doing anything.")

DOCTOR: Is that the kind of trouble you have, Mr. D?

MR. D: Sometimes I have trouble too, I don't know what I do.

MISS Q: How long has it been going on?

MR. D: Sometimes I feel all right.

MISS Q: How long have you been sick then? Do you have nightmares? I do. Do you have nightmares, you know, bad dreams?

MR. D: Yes. (Says he had a dream about death.)

DOCTOR: You dreamed that you saw yourself dead, or someone

else dead?

MR. D: I say I was dreaming, I don't know what I was doing.

DOCTOR: I see.

MISS N: 'Cause I'm going to tell you, doctor, I'm afraid of dead people.

DOCTOR: You're afraid of dead people?

MISS N: I'm afraid to die, and I'm not going to tell no stories about it, because ever since I took that dose of medicine that made me feel so bad, I've been living in a constant fear, something is going to happen to me.

MISS T: I know that I will have to die sometime, so what gives?

DOCTOR: Yes, how about that, why are you afraid to die?

MISS N: I don't know. It's just one of them things, that's all.

MR. E: I think most people are afraid of dying because of pain or of how they are going to die. If everyone knew how they were going to die they wouldn't be afraid. Some people are even afraid to go to funerals. But I think the biggest fear of death is how you're going to die. Some people die a tragic death. Some people die in their sleep, they don't feel nothing. I think some people fear the pain more than the death.

(Borderline cases often express a concern with and fear of death.)

DOCTOR: Are you afraid of dying, Mrs. Da?

MRS. Da: If it's about that dream, I don't know, because it was a long time ago that I dream. I had one or two bad dreams, then I wake up from my bed, I wake up in my living room and I took my children and so I was sure this was a dream—I can't be sure, because sometimes, especially when I'm nervous, I can't sleep and I need sleep—that's about it.

MRS. I: Sometimes, not really bad, they go away because when I wake up in the morning I don't remember what I had dreamed anyway.

MRS. Da: You forget your dreams? Not me.

MR. N: Doctor, I always dream of cowboys. When I was a kid—doctor, that's the only time I was happy, when I was a little kid.

Miss Q: How many days a week do you come here?

Mr. N: I come here every day. Nine years I've been coming here straight. On and off—and sometimes I get nervous and I feel like to punch the walls. You can't control me, you know. And then you drink beer, you go crazy sometimes.

Doctor: Do you drink, Mr. D? You don't drink beer?

Miss Q: I do.

Doctor: Do you drink beer, Mr. E?

Mr. E: Yes, but I don't like it.

Doctor: What do you drink?

Mr. E: Whiskey.

Doctor: It's not good for your brain, you know. (This positive statement is an example of the way the therapist must take a stand from time to time against self-destructive behavior that patients show. He continues along this line in the next intervention. He does not push the patient, however, in the following exchanges; having delivered his message, he withdraws to observe the reactions.)

Mr. E: I never went into a rage unless somebody made me mad—otherwise it doesn't affect my brain.

Doctor: It's not good for your brain, it kills brain cells.

Mr. E: I guess eventually I'll go crazy.

Miss T: Everybody says insane people get violent.

Mr. E: I'm not violent. If somebody did something to make you mad or offend you, you'd strike back, wouldn't you? I wouldn't say that's violent.

Miss T: I'll do that for kicks. If I have to do it, I mean naturally it would be for a good reason.

Mr. E: You take self-preservation—you protect yourself—you just don't go along and strike at guys.

Miss T: I know karate and judo.

Mr. E: It won't do you no good 'cause you're a woman. What would you do if a man my size attacked you? Are you going to use karate?

Miss T: Two weeks ago it saved my life.

Mr. E: But suppose the man knows the same things you do? or the man is stronger than you?

Miss T: I didn't give the man a chance. I put my bag down, and went like that, you know, real hard, and then I ran.

Miss Q: We won't be meeting on the twenty-fourth. Will we have another day instead?

Doctor: We just won't meet that day. I think we'll meet the thirty-first, though.

(Interventions like this are essential to clarify the time and place of the group meetings and to keep the therapy running smoothly. When the therapist misses appointments or fails to notify patients in advance that he will not be present, he is in need of supervision or should take a vacation. Perhaps both.)

Miss Q: Do you think it would be a good idea if I started to work full time? (The transference aspect of Miss Q's question is obvious. The therapist avoids joining her in a transference acting out by referring her question to the group. Her passive-aggressive demanding style is frustrated. As the discussion develops, it becomes apparent that any literal reply by the therapist to this question would have been irrelevant. Miss Q had already committed herself to go to work the following Monday.)

Doctor: Well, I don't know—let's see what the group thinks. Do you think she should work full time?

Mr. E: If she wanted to, I would. I would if I didn't have to come here.

Miss Q: I can get time off to come here.

Mr. E: Well, if you have to come here on that day—

Miss Q: Mr. V, do you think Miss Q should work full time?

Mr. V: If she wants to.

Miss Q: It's not a question of my wanting to, because I want to. It's a question of can I do it, because I have anxiety all day. I've been offered a job as public relations secretary at a hospital, but that would be too much pressure. And then I was offered a job in the office full time.

Mr. N: Ten-thirty to twelve is all right. It keeps you busy. You see, I don't know your name.

Miss T: (Tells her name.)

Doctor: Mr. D, do you think Miss Q should go back to work full time? Did you hear what she said?

MR. D: I hear what she said.

DOCTOR: Well, maybe it will get better.

MISS Q: Could I get worse if I work full time?

DOCTOR: What do you think, Mr. V? Do you think she will get worse if she works full time?

MR. V: Well, she should know how far she can go.

DOCTOR: Mr. E, do you have any ideas about it?

MR. E: I think it's entirely up to her.

DOCTOR: Miss N?

MISS N: I think the same thing. If she thinks it will do her more harm she better not do it.

MRS. Da: I agree with her.

MR. N: I agree with that.

MISS Q: I have to go on Monday. I have eight hours facing me this week. I think it will drive me crazier than I am.

MR. E: You know what I think you should do?

MISS Q: What?

MR. E: Like you figure you got those eight hours for a whole week—

MISS Q: Take one day at a time?

MR. E: When you go to work each morning, think about the money you're going to make and forget about the eight hours.

MISS Q: That's what prompted me to start to work full time— money. I've had a desire to do things that I didn't do for the past two years, now I feel like having money. I'm not making any, hardly. I make thirty-two dollars a week after they take off my social security.

MR. E: You can go downtown and see a nice show that you want, buy nice clothes, and you get to thinking about that, and thinking about the money—forget about those eight hours.

MISS Q: I have to get my teeth fixed.

MR. E: So worry about that, and don't worry about the eight hours.

MISS Q: I'm going to try it, because I don't think I can work part-time.

DOCTOR: Do you think Mr. D should go to work? You said before that you thought you might go to work; I wonder if he thought you should go to work? You said before that you should go to work (the therapist indicates various patients. He takes Miss Q's question about herself and asks it of her about another patient. This encourages her to look at the question a little more objectively and brings Mr. D into the discussion. It leads the patients to compare themselves with one another.)

Mr. D: It depends how I feel sometimes.

Doctor: Well, what do you think—let's hear what she thinks about it.

Miss Q: Well, not if he gets spells and loses contact with things, if he loses contact with reality and don't know what you're doing, I don't think so. Do you have a lot of fears?

Mr. D: Sometimes I walk and I hear a noise and I get scared and sometimes I don't hear anything and I'm not scared.

Doctor: Did you ever have that happen to you, Mr. E?

Mr. E: I'm afraid no, I'm scared of nothing. I got that way when I was in the Marines.

Doctor: Are you scared, Miss N?

Miss N: Yes, I am.

Doctor: You're not, Mrs. Da?

Mrs. Da: No.

Mr. N: Sometimes I am. I have nightmares when I sleep and when I get up I say "Mama, Mama," but she's dead. A cold fear comes and I get up out of bed. It happened a few times. But what about them though, why?

Doctor: What do you think, Miss T?

Mr. N: I'm all alone, that's why.

Miss T: Well, I guess it's the way you say.

Doctor: Well, why do you think he's scared the way he is?

Miss T: Because he's looking for something that doesn't exist.

Mr. N: Yes, when they leave you alone it's no good. Now I got to live by myself. My people went home, I've got to stay home like a jerk like that. I put on the television, and nothing happens. Then I go to bed and something happens.

Miss Q: I'd rather be alone. When someone invites me to a party or something, I dread it, I dread going there in my condition.

Doctor: How do you feel about being alone, Mr. E?

Mr. E: Well, about three years ago, I was in service and the only thing I was scared of was getting shot. Anything that moved, I shot at it, but so far as being alone, it doesn't bother me. If you've been in the service you find a lot of times you're alone for days. You've got to get used to it. Now, like in this case, I think I've seen men that have no family that live by themselves, that have, you know, they're just really alone, so they go to the park, they feed the pigeons, or they go to the zoo, you know? They do things to amuse themselves. Because you can sit in a place and amuse yourself. Some people take up knitting or putting puzzles together just to keep their mind occupied.

Doctor: Mr. V, do you have any ideas about this? Mr. D, how do you feel about being alone?

Mr. D: I can't answer this question.

Doctor: Do you ever spend much time by yourself?

Mr. D: Sometimes I . . . (mumbles)

Doctor: You what? You spent time by yourself?

Miss Q: When you have bad dreams for about two years and they start to increase in like color and thoughts and everything, does that mean you're getting better? Or does that mean you're getting worse?

Doctor: What do you say, Miss T?

Miss T: (Can't be heard because Mr. N speaks at the same time)

Doctor: You think it's getting worse, Mr. N?

Mr. N: Well, I stay with my friend; her name is D, and she says sometimes when you're lonely come and spend a couple of hours with me, to have coffee, and you forget about it and then you go to your room and read a book. That's a good idea. You read a book like you said, do a jigsaw puzzle.

Miss Q: I can't concentrate.

Mr. N: Dominos, you know.

Miss Q: Scrabble?

Mr. N: Yes, like he says. It's a good idea.

Docter: Why do you shake your head, Miss N?

Miss N: I'm shaking my head because I'm a person who has

fears and afraid to be alone and somebody can't come and tell me that nothing ain't going to bother you and come drink coffee with me. All right, that's okay for their house, but I've got to go back to my house. I don't live with them, so I don't see how drinking a cup of coffee with a neighbor and whatnot is going to help you get out of the scared feeling you're in. If you're afraid, you are just afraid, and by going to another house to amuse yourself ain't going to help any when you have to go back by yourself.

Miss Q: Are you afraid to go out of the house? Take a subway? Things like that?

Miss N: No, I'm not afraid to catch the subway, but just lately here I've been, for the past two or three weeks, I've been afraid, just about to do everything for myself.

Miss T: Tell me, did you ever have crank phone calls?

Mr. N: No.

Miss T: Every day I receive crank phone calls.

Miss Q: Have the number changed. Tell the telephone company.

Miss N: Have your number changed, that's all.

Mr. N: Sometimes they put a handkerchief over the phone, and they imitate like a girl. Maybe it could be a girl talking. Sometimes it does happen. Years ago there was a picture of a vampire.

(At this point the group interaction has become established.)

* * *

(The talk turned to television and horror movies. One patient had called "Frankenstein and all that" ridiculous.)

Doctor: (To Mr. E) Do you think Frankenstein and all that is ridiculous?

Mr. E: Entirely.

Doctor: Miss N, what do you think?

Miss N: I don't look at all that stuff. I dream too bad.

Doctor: What do you think, Mr. V?

Mr. V: It's a fantasy.

Doctor: Mrs. Da?

Mrs. Da: Not me. I don't dream about ghosts. A long time

ago I was scared about myself, about five years ago, but now I feel like some people—just nervous anyway, especially I have my first boy in Vietnam, and when I think of him I know that he has to come back alive. Whenever I think of him I say he has to come. I am scared of a lot of things, about my children. I have a lot of children; I have ten children. A long time ago I cared just about my husband—because he drinks too much. When I took my sickness, I was sure it came from my husband—because I have a job and I have to make everything for the house. But now a couple of years ago when my son joined the Marine Corps—well, I have a fate, you know my faith is like especially tonight—well, I don't know what it is with these people—I think about myself. I can't control myself. I think the other people the same thing. I'm scared of nothing because tonight I wake up in my bed and see my boys; I go to the bedroom, my living room. A long time ago—you see that coat is red, when I seen it I was scared. I prayed—I was thinking about this blood—but not now. Now I feel something special—like cold in my hands.

MR. N: Maybe it's the way you sleep. Do you sleep like this?

MISS Q: (To Mr. N) I wish you'd say something profound. What's your problem, that way you can't say I'm just looking at you.

DOCTOR: What do you think about what Mrs. Da just said?

MISS Q: I really didn't understand it too well. I heard her say something about the coat, it reminded her of blood and she used to be scared and she used to—I don't know.

DOCTOR: Miss N, what do you think about what Mrs. Da just said?

MISS N: I don't understand it too well.

DOCTOR: Mr. E, you understood it, didn't you? What do you think about it?

MR. E: I don't know.

DOCTOR: Mrs. I?

MRS. I: (This reply was not recorded well enough to be transcribed.)

MRS. Da: No, I wasn't talking about that. I was talking about any person has to be controlled by himself, right? I believe in

God, right? Well, some people don't care. We have to make a special thing of ourself. If I have to do everything, I control myself, I think I do.

DOCTOR: You have to take care of all ten children by yourself?

MRS. DA: Yes. Nine.

MISS Q: Don't the older ones take care of the little ones?

MRS. DA: Right now they do.

MISS Q: I used to live with a woman who had ten children. It was a mad house.

MRS. DA: But now my trouble comes from my husband because he drinks too much and he can't control himself. Sometimes I was in bad condition. I was nervous and I was crying, but I looked to my faith because it helped me. I think each one may control herself. Because if I want to cry I cry now. If I say no, I'm not going to do because it's no good in front of these people.

* * *

MISS Q: When I feel miserable, I go to work. Either that or I gulp down sleeping pills to escape the whole day.

DOCTOR: You don't drink any beer or any whiskey?

MISS Q: Maybe if I go out. I drink beer, yes. But not too much. If I go out on a weekend with my girlfriend, if I go shopping on Fifth Avenue in Brooklyn, I will stop in for a drink—martini.

DOCTOR: What do you think of this, Mr. E? (Mr. E's problems about drinking are turned around so he is asked to look at them in terms of someone else. This encourages him to a self-inspection by proxy.)

MR. E: Well, it's the same way when you're feeling bad, you're depressed. Some people are going to take a drink. I like his ideas when he said he would take a walk, because I got that way at one time three years ago. My kid was born in this hospital here and she had yellow jaundice. The doctor didn't know whether she was going to live. I left the hospital and I walked to Manhattan. I didn't take no drink, no nothing, just kept walking. I got over to Manhattan, I grabbed a subway, went home and went to bed. So sometimes walking helps, sometimes drinking helps, sometimes sleeping helps. I don't think—I'm not too much on drinking your problems away because I have tried that once before and I found out you can drink an excess amount, knock yourself out, go to sleep. It's like I said before, you wake up and you've got the same problems, and a headache.

Miss Q: You can escape from it temporarily by taking some pills and going to sleep.

Miss T: Temporarily you can.

Miss N: It helps you more than drinking can.

Miss Q: I would take pills every day. You get rid of one day at a time. You have nothing to do the whole day. You don't want to do anything.

Mr. N: Take Marilyn Monroe, she took an overdose. They all take them.

(All talking)

Mrs. Da: I want to ask this question. When we want to help a neighbor, I think this is a love.

Mr. E: Like you go to a neighbor and tell him you help him out. If they don't have food and you have food, you give them some food. To call the doctor for them.

Mrs. Da: Exactly.

Mr. E: Or to call the doctor?

Mrs. Da: Exactly.

Mr. E: But some people don't appreciate it.

Mrs. Da: Some people say love is just for a man or woman.

Mr. E: Love doesn't mean just for a man or woman. You can have a dog, you can love a dog.

Mrs. Da: Exactly.

Mr. E: You can love money, you can love clothes.

Mrs. Da: I think if everybody who have to love—especially to love cars. I can love everything of my people, and race and color. I love my neighbors, Italian, American, any kind. And I think any people need something special from us, right?

Mr. E: You need from each other. Let's say you're in this apartment, you've got neighbors all around, and if you want to be by yourself and one day you get sick and you can't get to the phone, if you socialize with your neighbors they come and help you, to call for you.

MRS. Da: That's right.

(The patients have begun to think about their positive feelings toward other people. This obviously relates to the way they can work with one another in the psychotherapy group.)

* * *

MISS Q: Do you think this group is too large?

DOCTOR: I don't know. Do you think it's too large, Miss Q?

MISS Q: Yes. (Miss Q's harping negative transference-resistance is expressed in this pseudorealistic objection to the presence of the other patients. She uses every excuse to complain or demand.)

DOCTOR: Do you think it's too large, Mr. V? Mr. D, do you think this group is too large? Do you think there are too many people here?

MR. N: No.

MR. D: It's not too many for me.

DOCTOR: How about you, Mrs. Da? (Mrs. Da had been talking to another patient in Spanish.) Why don't you tell what Mrs. D. is saying?

MRS. Da: I want to help a person out—she says she wants to know. Now she feels there is too much pain in the head. She has to buy the umbrella. She takes a pill, she feels a little better. She says it was raining.

DOCTOR: What do you think, do you think she should get an umbrella?

MRS. Da: It's a joke.

DOCTOR: Do you think she will learn to speak English?

MRS. Da: No.

DOCTOR: Do you think we should keep her in this group?

MRS. Da: She wants to know should she bring an interpreter?

DOCTOR: Well, tell her we will give her another appointment with a doctor and she can bring an interpreter.

(Spanish conversation)

DOCTOR: One at a time please. We can't all speak at once. Tell her we'll give her an appointment with another doctor and she can bring an interpreter. And tell her to learn to speak English too. You'll be taken care of, but come with an interpreter next time. (Patients who are obviously unsuited for group psychotherapy for any reason can directly but gently and firmly be removed. When possible, arrangements for alternative kinds of treatment should be provided.)

MRS. DA: Sometimes I feel a pain right here, in my throat. When I feel like that I go to bed. I take ten or fifteen minutes of sleeping and I feel fine.

DOCTOR: You lie down.

MRS. DA: Exactly. But I can't do this. I have a lot of children. When I lay down, I sleep about one minute or five minutes and it's better for me, but if there is noise it's no good for me.

DOCTOR: I guess we should all learn Spanish since she won't learn English.

MISS N: I'm too old to learn Spanish now.

DOCTOR: How old are you?

MISS N: Thirty-two.

DOCTOR: Then I don't stand a chance.

MISS Q: Will I be given individual therapy?

DOCTOR: Do you know what she's talking about, Mrs. Da?

MISS Q: I had a doctor here. I saw him for about a year and a half, and I was making a lot of progress and then he went on leave of absence and I've been stranded since July without a doctor, except for medication. I can go to a general practitioner and tell him what I want and he'll give it to me.

DOCTOR: Suppose we just stop. We'll meet again next Friday at ten-thirty. But the following Friday, the twenty-fourth, the clinic will be closed, but we will be open the thirty-first.

MRS. DA: We have to come every week?

DOCTOR: Every week.

(All talking at once.)

DOCTOR: Save it until next Friday.

*   *   *

The group ends on a note of resistance from Miss Q. The time of the next group session is explicitly announced. The requirement that the patients attend every Friday for this once a week group is made clear. Since a session is going to be missed on account of a holiday, patients are told this in advance as early as possible.

THE THIRD MEETING OF A NEW GROUP

To illustrate further the events of the first few sessions, the following excerpts from the third session of a new group of private patients in a psychiatrist's office are presented. The group consists of six young men diagnosed as ambulatory schizophrenics and borderline cases. The patients had all previously undergone individual psychotherapy. One had been treated in another group. One new patient was introduced at the beginning of this session. The other five had started in the group together.

These patients had been selected for group psychotherapy as a group of borderline and psychotic patients. That they were all male had more to do with the communicative aspects of the group than a selection on the basis of gender.

(Doctor introduces Mr. B to the group. Mr. B's arrival is ignored, like the arrival of an unwanted sibling.)

MR. B: I don't think I remember all your names.

MR. X: Well, I don't remember yours.

MR. H: (To Mr. X) You made an interesting remark last time. You said basketball was childish or not adult. I can't follow that train of thought. Why do you draw such a line?

MR. S: He meant it as when you're in your teens, that's a big thing, that's secondary, or even less. There are things other than that in life.

MR. P: There are so-called adult responsibilities, such as making a living, raising a family, et cetera, so that you can't clutch to that, so to speak. Whereas this was very important, you can get by with in an adolescent society. You can get by with it in an adult society. At one time it was very important, it was a reason for existence, but I did not. So in a way, I look back and say it was very childish, perhaps I should have been doing other things.

MR. H: What are you doing now to find reasons for existence?

(These patients all had identity problems. For them the reasons for living were not clear.)

Mr. P: I have reasons, but I don't know if they jell with reality as of the moment. It all depends on certain intangibles.

Mr. H: Did you say you weren't working?

Mr. P: Weren't working.

Mr. H: Living at home?

Mr. P: Living at home.

Mr. S: Do you want to get a job?

Mr. P: In a way I do. In another way I don't. In a way, I worked a couple of years ago. I went out and got a job as a messenger. I had two weeks of it and I figured that was enough after a two-year layoff, two weeks' work; when the third year is up, maybe I'll go back for a couple of more weeks. I mean, it's necessary, work, if you can get it, and you can get it if you try.

Mr. S: Why don't you want to work, though? Are you too lazy?

Mr. P: It isn't that I'm too lazy. It's that I have a great deal of difficulty in meeting people, and I shiver at the thought of riding in a subway.

Mr. H: I know someone, a daughter of a family I know, that has the same thing. She's scared to go anywhere alone, et cetera.

(At this point no intervention from the therapist is necessary to keep the interaction going. The mutual self-inquiry is going along, catalyzed by the group setting.)

Mr. P: If I go out at night, at midnight, and go to a saloon, I'm not afraid of nothing, I'll ride a bus or do anything. It depends on the goal, you see. In a way, to ride on the train and go to work is perfectly normal, and yet, somehow, I rebel against the very idea of it. I don't know, one of the big mistakes I made is in withdrawing from society. That's why, in a way, you have a certain advantage in that you are still within society.

Mr. H: Are you doing anything to get back into it?

Mr. P: Well, I have a project which I hope will pay off, so to speak. I don't know as yet whether it will or not. And I'm trying to pursue it to its logical conclusion. In fact, I have bet my life on it, so that it's one of those things I'm saying, if I can do this, why should I go to work like normal people; see?

Mr. X: Are you inventing something?

MR. P: No; writing. It's kind of strange. I don't know, I have had very little encouragement.

MR. S: What are you writing about?

MR. P: I usually write about people and what they're doing, you know. I don't know, it's a very complex thing. It's hard to get into. It's about a basketball player, incidentally. It's a basketball player who attaches his reasons for existence to basketball.

MR. H: You're writing about yourself.

MR. P: No. In a way, I would say the personality is me, but the circumstances are fictional, which is usually the case in the first book you ever write.

MR. H: And you figure if that book succeeds it will be a best seller and the money will roll in and you won't have to work?

MR. P: Not only assume it will be a best seller. I expect to win a Nobel Prize many, many years from now.

MR. X: Are you kidding or are you serious?

MR. P: No, I'm saying if I'm going to bet my life on it, I might as well go whole hog.

MR. H: What will you do if the first one doesn't succeed?

MR. P: I don't really know. I'll probably cry, I guess.

MR. X: I'll have to defend the arts and say that's a terrible goal in literature, trying to get a Nobel Prize.

MR. P: I'm not interested in that particularly.

MR. X: I am.

MR. P: I'm saying I will write and let us hope I will win such awards.

MR. S: So you won't have to work like someone else in an office?

MR. X: You didn't *say* that.

MR. P: I said if I have to do it, I might as well win the Nobel Prize.

MR. H: And after awhile you might like writing so much that—

MR. P: I do enjoy writing. It demands a great deal of you. You put a great deal of work into it, you want some remuneration for it, and as yet I have had none.

MR. H: A lot of writers never did, for a long time.

MR. P: But they usually have something else going for them.

Mr. X: You seem to want money.

Mr. P: Not particularly.

(The spontaneous interaction continues. Although the group is only in its third session, the selection of patients has been such that the group interaction goes almost by itself.)

Mr. X: When you say you're basing your whole life on this, what are you going to live on? It sounds very unrealistic.

Mr. P: It's unrealistic, but at the same time I'm aware of the fact that writing can be quite rewarding, financially speaking.

Mr. H: I think it's better than just sitting at home and rocking in a rocking chair and pretending to be Jack Kennedy. (This session occurred in early 1962.) Of course, again, I have always been interested in writing, et cetera, and I admire what you are doing. (Mr. H is curious about the blatant ambition of Mr. P to become great. Mr. H has also been ambitious, a secret admirer of German militarism, but has assumed the role of a quiet, studious clerical person.)

Mr. P: I don't know, I've spent six years at it and I've completed my novel and I'm rewriting it, and I'm very pleased with it. My own critical sense tells me this is very good.

Mr. S: Did anyone else ever read the book?

Mr. P: No, I haven't got it completed yet. I've completed it, but I'm in the stage of rewriting.

Mr. N: If you come to the realization that writing were a dead-end wall, would it make it any easier or help you in any way to go out and get a job?

Mr. P: I think it would be a crushing defeat, since I have tended to identify with my work. This is something I've done.

Mr. N: Well, let's assume for some reason, other than the success or failure of this particular book, you couldn't write.

Mr. P: What would I do otherwise?

Mr. N: If this demand which you feel is made on you were not made, would this have any effect on your ability to go out and look for a job?

Mr. P: What prevents me more than anything else are certain ideas I attach to getting a job.

Mr. N: What does getting a job mean? (Mr. N is really very

concerned about himself. He wonders what kind of work he is going to do.)

MR. P: Coming in contact with people.

MR. N: You do already come into contact with people. You go to a tavern, and so forth.

MR. P: Very rarely do I go to a tavern nowadays. I don't have any money.

MR. N: You did in the past. Wasn't that one of the reasons, meeting people?

MR. P: I used to enjoy meeting people, but since I've gotten this bee in my bonnet about writing, I look at myself as a failure.

MR. N: You enjoyed meeting people before you got this bee in your bonnet. If this bee were out of your bonnet, then you might enjoy meeting people again?

MR. P: But I have a case of not accepting myself, as looking upon myself as defeated, and I say I have to wrest victory from—

MR. N: Do you really think that it's meeting the people that makes it difficult for you to go and find a job?

MR. P: That, more than anything, I'm afraid.

MR. H: When we first came here, I thought you were more or less a fellow that knew what it was all about, your manner of speaking. Maybe, again, when I look at you and I sort of generalize, I think, he's a little, fat, happy-go-lucky fellow. (Here Mr. H comes out of his shell to cut down Mr. P.)

MR. P: I tended to be that. I led a very active life, but somehow I withdrew. I was very active, and I can't see myself in this sensitive art and the ivory tower. It's against my nature, in a way. I want writing to be a confirmation of life, not a denial of it.

MR. H: Besides writing, are you doing anything just to get out and meet people more, and so on?

MR. P: No.

MR. H: Because the writing may be an excuse to retire more and more.

MR. P: It is a kind of excuse, but the strange thing is I find the writing becoming now more practical. It's as though as I come nearer to reality, it's the writing, and at one time I was very much removed from it. The writing has kept alive my personality. Otherwise, it would have shriveled up and just collapsed. This is five years I have been away from people.

MR. H: Do you find this group helpful in terms of meeting people?

MR. P: I find that it is. For example, the other goup (this patient had been previously treated in another group), it would take me a long time to get into the group, and I was very hostile, whereas, within this group, I don't seem to have any hostility towards any one of you as of the moment. I feel better with you in the beginning than with the other group at the beginning.

MR. N: Just a while ago you said you didn't like to look at yourself as the ivory-tower artist. Three weeks ago, the first time we were talking, you felt you were somehow altogether detached from society and felt a very great responsibility. Both of these things you said you don't like, and then you said that you're betting your life on this.

(Mr. N points out the contradictions in Mr. P's statements. This encourages Mr. P's self-examination. Mr. N follows Mr. H's lead in challenging Mr. P. Mr. P's grandiosity can be effectively deflated by such exchanges as this without his losing the support he needs. Mr. H and Mr. N will stop or the therapist will intervene if Mr. P shows signs of being harmed by these attacks.)

MR. P: That responsibility, I think I was saying this: That I used to feel very responsible, you know, tending to identify with society, and, therefore, anything in society which is bad, I'm in some way responsible. I've removed that.

MR. N: Aren't these things somehow connected? That is, the ivory-tower writing and social responsibility? Don't they have a relationship?

MR. P: They did at the time, and when I first wrote I found I was a moralist, saying this is wrong, this is right, and now I've become amoral.

MR. N: Do you still consider yourself an ivory-tower artist?

MR. P: I kind of look at myself as caged, and the cage is anxiety and fear, and so I'm in the cage, I might as well do something. I might as well do this to sort of educate myself, to take advantage of the thing. I realize that part.

MR. N: That's why you write. But it doesn't answer the question. What kind of an artist are you? You say you're caged and you've got to do something so you write. My question was, insofar as you said that you didn't like the idea of being an ivory-tower-type artist, since you are caged, you must be some kind of writer; what kind of writer is that?

(Mr. P has defended himself and presented some of his most troublesome feelings to the group.)

MR. P: You mean what would be the nature of my writing?

MR. N: Is it something other than ivory tower?

MR. P: Now you're getting into a question of what is an ivory-tower artist.

MR. N: You seemed to know what that meant when you said it.

MR. P: I meant someone who goes off by himself and shuts his eyes to the world and sort of dedicates himself to the purity of art.

MR. N: You're not doing that?

MR. P: No. For me art is a means, not an end.

MR. N: But you're shut off from the world by a cage.

MR. P: I feel that way. I feel as though I'm in prison, somehow.

MR. N: Is this a difference between you and an ivory-tower artist?

MR. P: I'm very much aware of reality because it upsets me.

MR. X: What upsets you?

MR. P: Reality. I don't like the reality that I'm broke, no money, more or less friendless. In any way I look at myself, I have to turn thumbs down and say, you're just a one hundred percent washout. I'm very much aware of this apparent failure on my own part.

MR. X: You say you don't like the fact that you're broke, but you won't go out and get a job?

MR. P: Yes, but somehow it doesn't seem connected, as though my prime object is not money.

MR. N: Is one of the prime factors in the sense of your being a washout, money?

MR. P: Yes. It's as though I say, other people judge you by

how much money you make, how much I make. I'm not making money, therefore, I'm nothing.

MR. X: You sit here and tell me you're not a part of it and away from it all, but every time it comes to make a judgment of value or worth, you always seem to say something that, in effect, is saying it's the other people who won't think this, or I won't look good in other people's eyes. I don't think that you're really being correct when you say you're not a part of it.

MR. P: My awareness of other people is very important and I don't want to be that way. I don't want to be a slave of your opinion, and yet, I am. If you know what I mean.

(Mr. P expresses his dilemma very directly. To him, to be the slave of opinion is to assume an identity. This is a terrifying prospect to him.)

MR. X: Then you're very much a part of what goes on around you.

MR. P: I want to be detached from your view, in a way that I don't like the idea that meeting you I'm going to try to be very likeable. I would like to be myself and hope that being around myself, because in doing that I implicitly condemn myself in saying: If you knew the real me, you wouldn't like me.

MR. H: Doesn't this go back to the basic idea that you don't like yourself as you are? It's not so much what other people think of you that matters, but you hate you.

MR. P: Yes. I don't accept myself. At one time I did accept myself, and because I accepted myself I expected other people to accept me. Now because I'm condemning myself, I expect other people to do it.

MR. H: Right. And so you're scared.

MR. P: I say, let me get away from people, because I don't want to be condemned.

MR. N: Does your being yourself mean having money?

MR. P: I would like to have money. I'm not opposed to the idea.

MR. N: You can't go out and get money because you're a slave to your opinions?

MR. P: I don't know. It's as though I want to avoid you. It's as though I want to avoid you. It's as though people threaten me, that the best thing to do is stay away from people. (Mr. P's fear of conformity or assuming his identity is expressed directly.)

Mr. H: Again, did you have any specific thoughts about what individuals in this group thought of you? For example, myself. Have you thought what I think of you or is it too early in the game? (This patient is making a great effort to make the group psychotherapy work for him. It is one of the few opportunities he has ever had to speak frankly and openly with his peers.)

Mr. P: The first few meetings I attended with this group, I tended to judge myself well, in saying that I have an advantage over them in that I have the experience in the other group. But I have been thinking to myself, as *you* gather more experience, I gather less and less in this group. And I'm saying to myself, the more you know about it, the more I will sink into the background and sit here and listen to you.

Mr. H: What about the idea that we might want to help you?

Mr. P: I don't know, it's as though if I keep silent you can't really help me. I can defeat you that way.

Mr. H: We won't let you keep silent.

Mr. P: You can keep silent. You say, "I don't know," and push people away.

Mr. H: Then you defeat yourself.

Mr. P: I know. And you ask yourself, why do you do it?

Mr. H: Then later on you kick yourself for having done it.

Mr. P: Yes. Very often—I don't know how *you'll* react during the course of the treatment—very often I go out and say, why do I sit there? I have so many things to say. Why didn't I say them? (The patient's doubts about the treatment are expressed. It is very important that this occur at the beginning and be recognized as it comes up throughout the treatment.)

Mr. H: Well, I find myself doing that now. Again, it's easy for me to say. I don't have your fears to that sense or that degree.

Mr. P: To me it's a crippling thing.

Mr. H: And I wonder what's the solution, what's the key? But also I wonder, what are you doing? I look at myself—in other words I'm going to night school, and this can serve as a good ex-

cuse for not going out too much, that I'm devoting a lot of time to
libraries and working on papers. But I realize it and I date and
I square dance, and to me, square dancing is a big thing in my life.
This gives me an out and a chance to meet people, and so forth
and so forth. And I wonder, what are *you* doing to meet people.

(The patients begin to discuss how they have been trying to
help themselves. This precedes their wondering how and if the
group psychotherapy will help.)

Mr. P: Not very much. I don't do anything.

Mr. H: *This* is something right now (indicating the group).

Mr. P: Yes. This has helped me.

Mr. X: Is that why you square dance, to meet people?

Mr. H: Yes. I enjoy doing it. It gives me exercise. I enjoy
doing it. As I said earlier, I don't drink or smoke. I don't like
going to a tavern or night clubs. If I weren't square dancing, it
would be social dancing. But I prefer the people at square dances.

Mr. X: What is social dancing?

Mr. H: The other places. I go to the "Y" or I go to Roseland,
but usually the "Y." The other places you have people drinking;
not that the "Y" crowd is that soft either.

Mr. S: People at the bar get more friendlier and are nicer to
be with.

Mr. H: Also, a church dance; but again, each to his own. But
again, do you have any skills? Or again, all right, the idea that
you like basketball because you could do it well, you could domi-
nate. I used to be the same way. I used to play baseball when I
was bigger than the other kids because I could do it better than
them, but when they got bigger than me, I hated baseball and I
quit. Again, do you have any other skills?

Mr. P: I don't have any other skills, unless it's the cue stick,
but I don't want to go back into the pool parlor.

Mr. H: Why don't you teach kids to play basketball?

Mr. P: No, I have given up basketball, for good reason: I
have deteriorated.

Mr. H: Well, again, I tell myself the same thing, why go for
treatment after treatment, where in many ways you've reached
the point of going out and doing something and changing. One of

my problems is I always look to somebody else to give me the solution to my problem. I have to do it myself.

Mʀ. X: Out doing what, do you know? (Mr. X does not understand exactly what the others have been talking about. He has listened carefully. Now he begins to try to learn, but he cannot avoid trying to impress and manipulate the other patients.)

Mʀ. H: I work in a bank. I don't like it. I could change or go to another bank or drop out of banking. But banking gives me the opportunity to go overseas. I can sit here and talk about it but until I try to go to the other bank, this solution to the problem won't be reached.

Mʀ. N: What prevents you from going to another bank?

Mʀ. H: I rationalize and say I want to finish my Master's degree first. But partly it is the idea I say I'm not good enough. Partly I can use the doctor as a rationalization, in that I can see the doctor on my lunch hour and with the other bank I wouldn't be able to do that. I throw up excuses.

Mʀ. P: Are you not doing the same thing I'm doing, in a way? I refuse to change my life because I'm afraid I won't get a job. In other words, I know I have to change and I know I have to do it, but I won't, and I rationalize it.

Mʀ. H: Yes.

Mʀ. P: In other words, we're discontent with our lives but we won't change. (Mr. P now scrutinizes Mr. H to the advantage of both.)

Mʀ. H: I mentioned in the last treatment with the doctor that I have no friends. I have met one or two people square dancing. But as far as friends after work to go play cards with or to go to a movie with, I don't have any. I have a girlfriend, but that's one person. And I tell myself: You ought to join another group or join Rotary, or some organization, and meet people. But I always say, when I get my Master's degree.

Mʀ. S: Does your girlfriend have friends?

Mʀ. H: Yes.

Mʀ. S: Don't you double-date with them?

Mʀ. H: No. I don't know why.

Mʀ. S: Do you find that you don't like the people? When you

first meet him, do you say I don't like him, I don't want to be his friend?

MR. H: A lot of people I don't like. I was in England for awhile. I kept thinking, English women are really women; there is no place like it. Then I say, quit kidding yourself, you don't want to go back to the English income. One of my buddies gets the English newspapers—there again, my buddy at work. After five it stops. Anyway, I see the newspapers and I tell myself, you don't want to go there. Here in New York I don't care for people. I don't care for the way they speak, and so on, but I'm still in New York, so I go around seeking something. Not really seeking; thinking about it. Until I actually get out and do, I'm still the same way. So I ask myself, again, as you say, there are certain similarities between you and me, and I sometimes think there are similarities between all of us. Earlier I was telling myself, I don't have the same problems these characters do; I don't take dope, I don't feel detached, this and that, but then again, there are similarities. (Mr. H begins to wonder why he doesn't like people.)

MR. N: What keeps you in New York?

MR. H: The idea of going overseas, the idea of trying the other bank, the idea of getting my Master's. New York isn't that bad. It was also the idea: Will I like another place better? Maybe I will and maybe I won't. I don't want to shift around all my life.

MR. S: What big goal do you have after you get your Master's?

MR. H: To get married. To me this is a big goal. But then to go overseas.

MR. S: Once you get your Master's you can go overseas?

MR. H: I could go overseas with the bank I'm in, but I don't like their salary.

MR. S: But you need a Master's to go overseas?

MR. H: No. I rationalize it that way. Another rationalization is, I've worked so long for my Master's I say if I go to the other bank they might say, we'll send you overseas in six months and if I say I want to finish my Master's they may say, we won't want you when *you* want to go. You have to go when we want.

MR. S: Did that girl that you're going out with become a problem in your life?

MR. H: No.

MR. S: When you met her, you weren't nervous and everything?

MR. H: When I first met her, yes. I think of marrying her once in awhile. When we talk about kids, she doesn't particularly care for kids. But I don't ditch her because I met her at a good time. We have similarities. And I found her the nicest thing that's come along in my life yet. If I give that up, there might not be anything else.

MR. S: I guess a lot of people think that.

MR. N: Having this understanding with yourself, if you can call things rationalizations, it doesn't allow you or help you in any way to overcome them?

(The self-presentation has continued. This expository activity has not required intervention by the therapist.)

MR. H: Yes. Actually a lot of the understanding I've only reached lately, thanks to the doctor. And I used to think, well, I'm not getting anything out of it, and it's been a long, slow process, and again, I feel there is a long way to go, in certain respects, until I start realizing a lot more things. But the things I've realized, I've realized within the past year. So I figure, all right, I only have till this September to get my Master's; I'll be through then. So I figure, why change everything now? Wait till then. This, again, may be a rationalization. (The transference aspect of this positive statement about the therapist is obvious. Mr. H was sincerely grateful, yet his attitude toward the therapist was distant, fearful, and suspicious. His parents were an unusual pair. His mother spoke of his father as being her inferior, yet never demonstrated any real evidence of her superiority. Mr. H had spent the first year of his life in a hospital because of some obscure feeding difficulty. His parents were strict disciplinarians toward him. They were never physically demonstrative of affection to one another or to the patient.)

MR. N: When you run into one of these problems and you recognize it as a challenge, is your reaction to it now what it was before you had the realization of rationalizing?

MR. H: No. Before, when I was faced with a problem, I would throw up my hands and quit and say, I can't possibly do that any-

way. I'm not good enugh. Now it's changed. I say, look, get hold
of yourself, you know you can do it, everyone else is doing it. Even
if you don't succeed, the idea that I've tried is important to me.
And the idea of succeeding is nice too, but the important idea is
that I tried instead of just throwing up my hands and quitting
and ducking and just going the other way, and so on.

MR. N: What in your mind prevents you from carrying this
thing over to the things you mentioned you want?

MR. H: Of trying, and so on? Well, I rationalize. Maybe the
idea it's been too recent to carry it over, but as long as I keep going
out with the girl I'm going out with now, and I've been dating her
a year, again, I tell myself the relationship is changing, maybe
she'll be more in favor of marriage as time goes on. And I should
have a serious talk with her. Am I wasting my time, or not? Because I'm having a good time. Even if I am wasting time, I'm
learning a lot of things. When the time comes to shift, it will be
that much easier.

MR. N: I was thinking more of the bank in Europe.

MR. H: I've lost the question.

MR. N: Why is it that you can't carry this "I'm going to try"
thinking over? (Mr. N is asking why he is unable to act according
to what he knows is best for himself.)

MR. H: Well, going back to the bank, I was a lending officer
assistant until recently. In our bank you can start off as a general
clerk or trainee, if you're a college graduate, and then you can become a lending officer assistant. Then the next job is just a glori-
fied clerk. I was an assistant for three years. I kept thinking one
of these days I'm going to dump the whole thing and go over to
(another bank) and get a good job, and so forth and so forth, and
even though I'm an assistant I can get more money and maybe get
to go overseas. And so, recently, they made me an officer, and so
now I can figure, well, I can't quit right after that. Couldn't he
handle it? And besides, I became an officer in October. Every
month I'm an officer I get more experience to sell myself. And
partly the idea I want someone else to make up my mind for
me. And the idea if I go to the other bank and don't go into
personnel administration, which interests me more than bank-

ing. But if I don't go over to the other bank—and this is the way it goes back and forth. I don't decide and I don't act. Now I figure, well, the time is coming when I have to act.

MR. N: Again, I want to talk about your concern with having tried.

MR. H: Why is this so important?

MR. N: Why is it that you can't carry over your thinking in this particular situation, which is very important to you?

(Mr. N won't let Mr. H evade the issue. This forces Mr. H to look at himself and indicates that Mr. N is scrutinizing himself. This kind of using a question about another patient repeatedly to maintain interest in a question raised by a patient about another but really about himself could not happen in individual psychotherapy. It happens regularly in group psychotherapy and serves to encourage the questioner to examine himself as well as the patient to whom the question is asked.)

MR. H: In terms of going to London?

MR. N: Whatever. In going to another bank and achieving the things you want to achieve and in other areas that you say is important. Why don't you carry that kind of thinking over?

MR. H: Maybe it's too big for me.

DOCTOR: Maybe he does, you know; he might.

MR. H: But I haven't.

DOCTOR: You might have been doing it.

MR. H: Going over to the other bank?

DOCTOR: No. It doesn't mean that you have to go to the other bank. It doesn't mean that you have to do anything. (Referring to carrying the thinking over into activity. It appeared that the discussion was at an impasse. It appeared important to support Mr. H at this point. He actually had carried into action a great many of his plans. Mr. N, on the other hand, had not faced directly the need to meet the requirements of his college courses. He had evaded his self-imposed requirements as well. At this point it appeared that he was apt to use Mr. H as his whipping boy.)

MR. H: You're losing me. Your question was, why don't I try in terms—

MR. N: My question was whether or not you knew why you didn't try to carry over your thinking in this particular situation.

DOCTOR: You're making two assumptions in that question. That he didn't try. He may be doing both, you know. You're making two assumptions in that question. (Deliberately pushing the question into another form. This enabled Mr. H to come up with a responsive answer with its transference identification with the aggressor, Mr. N, in his self-condemnation.)

MR. H: I hadn't tried going over to the other bank. Trying has become important, but it's only recently that I have realized that in practically everything I would try half-heartedly. If I succeeded, fine, but if I didn't, I wouldn't try any harder. I would say I'm no good and give up.

DOCTOR: What he's doing may be the best thing for him to do. That's a possibility, you see. (To Mr. N in support of Mr. H.)

MR. P: He seems to have good reasons for staying where he is. Once you get the Master's degree that should increase your value as an employee.

MR. H: Right, but in my present bank there is no good reason to stay, unless I can look ahead and say in my present bank I can get promotions quickly, compared to the other banks, and maybe become an assistant vice-president and sell my services. But by that time I'll be committed to banking and I won't have the opportunity to try another field if I want to. I figure banking where I am now is bad. I don't like it that much. I like the customer contact but I don't like working with balance sheets and figures. Therefore, if I go to the other bank where most of the figures and balance sheets are done by the lower echelon, I can have customer contact. Also, they will get me overseas in six months and if I don't like it in a year or two, I can try another field. Again, I figure I'll have good reasons until September, when I get my Master's. By that time I'll have eleven months' experience as an officer, I'll have my Master's, and I won't have a good excuse for staying where I am without trying (another bank), for example, or if that doesn't succeed, maybe trying my other field. I don't know, when September rolls around, I'll have to readjust a lot of things. (Mr. H's ambivalence about his career is a reflection of his identity problems.)

MR. X: Do you intend to stay in banking?

MR. H: That's my big problem. Sometimes I think yes, sometimes no.

MR. X: What are you going to get if you stay in banking?

MR. H: Let's say I'll go to the other bank. I'll make a good living; I might make above average income, especially if I went overseas. As far as satisfaction in terms of having accomplished something, I will have done the daily job, but not really done much good. My thinking is more in terms of social welfare, in terms of training people or helping people; something; teaching; the idea, if you teach, you've brought someone up a bit. I want to help people raise themselves. This, to me, is accomplishment.

MR. X: Raise themselves to what?

MR. H: To be better than they were before. (Here Mr. H's desire to help others and concern about the welfare of others is a reflection of the deprivations he has suffered and his wish that someone had been concerned about him and wanted to help him.)

MR. N: Would you explain a little more clearly what your objection was to the question? (Mr. N had been unaware of what he was doing. It appeared best to handle this question literally.)

DOCTOR: You assumed he didn't know what he was doing and he hadn't used it in any way.

MR. H: I didn't get that assumption.

DOCTOR: He made two assumptions in that question.

MR. N: I didn't understand it.

MR. H: Why is it so important?

DOCTOR: He was assuming that you hadn't used your capabilities in considering these problems that you have.

MR. H: That's exactly what he said. He said, why don't you carry this trying over—or whatever it is—into these problems that you bring up?

DOCTOR: And he assumed that you hadn't, when you might have been.

MR. N: I assumed that he hadn't because he said he hadn't gone to the other bank.

DOCTOR: Yes, I know. But the assumption is that unless he

goes to the other bank, then he's not doing anything. That's a false assumption. He may do things without going to the other bank.

MR. H: In terms of the bank problem?

DOCTOR: Yes.

MR. H: Or in terms of other problems?

DOCTOR: Well, whatever. It may not be appropriate to go to the other bank at this time anyway.

MR. H: Well, at least I take comfort that it isn't appropriate for me.

MR. X: I was going to say before, you gave about six reasons for not going to the other bank and after each one you said: This is a rationalization. I was going to ask you if you had a concrete reason or reasons that you thought were concrete why you didn't go. One of them you mentioned, but skipped over very quickly; you said perhaps they will send you overseas before you finish schooling. But then you talked about it a little more and built it into a rationalization. (Mr. X is probably right, but his reason for saying this is a part of his positive reaction to the therapist and his desire to help the therapist. Mr. X had probably the highest I.Q. in this group.)

MR. H: Again, in some ways I tend to look at many of my concrete reasons as being rationalizations, because from the past I have realized many of my ideas I have come up with were rationalizations.

MR. X: That's a pretty damn good reason, if they sent you over before you end your schooling.

MR. H: If in six months—and you take six months away from September you come to around April—so theoretically I should be going over there around April or May, but I have put it off until September.

DOCTOR: Mr. B, what do you think about all this? (This intervention was made to interrupt the flow of the discussion and to insure Mr. B of a chance to talk. He did not participate in this group session and soon dropped out of the group.)

MR. B: I don't know. I have been listening, but I just don't know what to say about it. I would like to listen a couple of more times, then maybe I can join in.

MR. H: We're still in the feeling around stage, actually. To-night represents the first real discussion of any real problems, or problems per se. The last two meetings we have been wonder-ing, What's this all about? What's in it for me? Can it do any good? etc. So don't feel too strange about it. (This represents a fair summary of the first sessions of this new psychotherapy group.)

MR. X: Have you ever been in a group before?

MR. B: No, I haven't.

MR. X: He's the only one who has, that fellow over there (indicating Mr. P). This is our third meeting, except for him. That expression you used, "selling your services," is that a bank-ing thing? (Mr. X had had some experiences as a male prostitute.)

MR. H: How do you mean?

MR. X: Is that a banking expression?

MR. H: It might be just from reading vocational literature or always trying to find the answer to what I really want to do. It might be because banking is pretty much price fixed, shall we say? The rates are pretty much the same, interest rates, and so on, so what do you have to sell? You have services. Again, I was with (an airline) as a registration clerk for awhile. There, again, whatever you are doing is service.

MR. X: Did you overbook any flights at all? (Mr. X lets the issue drop and changes the subject. He may have taken the expression as an idea of reference to his prostitution.)

MR. H: No. But there again, it was a low-paying job.

MR. S: How much was a low paying job?

MR. H: Two hundred a month net. And considering the fact that passengers ask you for information or flight bookings, you had to book them, it was your responsibility; if you messed them up some way, then they get mad at (the airline), and everything else. Also, actually, again, you start off as a sales agent 3. Then you go up to 2 and then 1. I was a sales agent 1 because I handled the night shift on two nights, Friday and Saturday nights midnight to eight in the morning, all by myself.

MR. S: All they gave you for that was fifty dollars a week?

MR. H: Right. My present job is low paying, as far as I'm concerned. I'm earning—well, it isn't important what I'm earning right now. But starting off, the bank starts a college graduate at 375 or 400. (Another bank) will start at 475 or 500.

MR. S: What's that come to a week?

MR. H: Well, a hundred a week gross, but, again, in our bank, the higher up you go, you're always losing out. All the higher ups are griping about low pay. To me it's not much money. Again, it's relative. What may be low pay to me might not be to you.

MR. S: That's why I asked you.

MR. H: But to me a thousand bucks a month is high pay, and I think it is to you, too.

MR. X: I can say a thousand dollars a month is high pay, but where you might consider four hundred dollars a month low, someone else might not.

MR. H: Yes. If I were in college getting a summer job, four hundred dollars a month would be fabulous. It's all relative. Again, sometimes I think money is the end all, and other times I think, why money? Because then you can go out and do a lot of good, aids to education, philanthropies, and so forth.

(The patients have been comparing what they want and what they think they can get. This reflects their own ideas of self-worth.)

MR. X: No, you can go out and have fun. If you're giving money to charity, why are you doing it? It's fun.

MR. H: Well, it depends on how you define fun. Then I think also if you're going to spend eight hours a day working—or seven hours, as is the case in New York—

MR. X: Five hours.

MR. H: —you might as well have fun doing it, and I'm not having fun. I'm getting a sense of accomplishment doing work. The sense of accomplishment lies in doing work, not the type of work I'm doing, if I make myself clear. If I write ten letters, fine, I have written ten letters and the work is done, but I don't get any sense of accomplishment out of the letters I've written. I don't see they're doing much good.

MR. X: What would give you a sense of accomplishment?

MR. H: Building people up, educating them, teaching; and then again, teaching doesn't pay enough.

MR. X: What are you going to do with all your money? Seriously, it doesn't pay enough, but what are you going to do with all this money?

MR. H: Save it, invest it, make more money, become a millionaire; go down in the history books as that, too. But money grows, a sense of building something, building money.

MR. S: You have no use for it? Maybe spending it.

MR. H: Not even spending it. You can spend only so much.

MR. X: That's disgusting.

MR. H: Beyond that it's a matter of making money and doing good with it or making it for the sheer challenge of making it.

MR. X: Doesn't it make you nauseous?

MR. H: No.

MR. X: It makes me nauseous because it's so purposeless; you build this pile of money, take hundred-dollar bills and wrap it in paper like in a bank, you can build card houses out of this money.

MR. S: Like Scrooge.

MR. H: But you can also use it for a lot of good, like college scholarships, Ford Foundations, Rockefeller Foundations, and so on. Maybe I've set my goal so high I say, what's the use of trying. (Mr. H's obsessive-compulsive trends with their reactive altruism are evident.)

MR. X: Then what's the use of trying for something less?

MR. H: Maybe just for the sense of accomplishment.

MR. S: Trying for something less, he can accomplish something less.

MR. H: Or you can start with less and go higher, build it up to more. It's the same thing with teaching, what do you start with?

MR. X: What do you end up with?

MR. H: If you're a good teacher you can end up with more and you have accomplished something. Then I wonder, why don't I go into teaching? It's nice vacations, but low pay. And I have the visions of getting overseas on the American income.

MR. X: Nice vacations, by the way, is a farce; you realize that, don't you?

Mr. H: On teachers? No, I don't realize it.

Mr. X: On educators, not teachers. There are teachers that teach certain months a year and take off the summer. Most of them do. But you want to be a teacher? You want to be an educator?

Mr. H: I don't know.

Mr. X: The way you're talking there is more to it than teaching.

(Identity problems continue to be discussed.)

Mr. H: Also I tell myself I don't want to go into a classroom and teach the same thing two hours a day, year after year, over and over.

Mr. X: There are schools that you can have different classes if you really want to. It seems really empty to me.

Mr. S: Today I realized the problem I had for a long time, that whenever I want something, like Monday is a holiday and there will be no work, and in other years it was a birthday or a vacation or something like that, and I feel that when I heard Monday I'd be off, I said to myself, that's no good for you, you'll probably get sick and you won't enjoy it and you'll be in the whole weekend. And when a birthday is close I feel, oh, shit, I'll die before my birthday comes. I wait for it as though something would happen and ruin it on me. (Mr. S, a simple schizophrenic, operated on a crude pleasure-seeking basis at times.)

Mr. H: Did something bad happen?

Mr. S: Not all the time. But I always used to have this feeling.

Mr. H: Every time I wanted to do something important, I said I'll probably get a cold, and nine times out of ten I did get it.

Mr. S: If I'm waiting to go out on a date, I start to think at the last minute she'll break it, or for some reason I won't be able to make it.

Mr. H: I used to think the same way, and then I start thinking, how often does it actually happen?

Mr. S: That's the way I think too.

Mr. X: Did you ever try to make it happen?

MR. S: No.

MR. H: I doubt that you would realize that you were making it happen.

MR. X: No, I agree.

MR. H: It might happen and you'll think, gee, what an accident.

MR. S: Like if I was going out with a girl I would try to make sure specifically nothing would happen.

MR. H: Depending upon thinking in terms of what you mean by nothing would happen. You might break an arm or a leg.

MR. X: I know a guy who was shipping out and it did happen, he broke a couple of toes. (Mr. X had had a great variety of experiences with several kinds of people. He frequently wanted to show that he was experienced and knowing.)

MR. S: Did he ship out anyway?

MR. X: Yes.

MR. H: Have you been in the service?

MR. X: No.

MR. S: I joined up with a couple of friends of mine. We're leaving on active duty. I'm supposed to leave the end of August.

MR. H: How long do you go for?

MR. S: Two years. I was told I could go where I want to.

MR. H: You'll have a ball.

MR. S: I hope.

MR. H: I used to think in basic training, will I survive? I'm not as strong as the other fellows. But I had a good time.

MR. S: I know you can't have a good time being in bed at nine and working and having some guy telling you what to do.

MR. X: You get used to it.

MR. H: The thing is, you can't fight the service. If you fight it, you'll end up in the stockade. Also, if you're in the stockade for six months, then you got to put in six months more when you are out.

MR. X: Really?

MR. H: Unless they give you a "D. D."

MR. X: What's that?

MR. H: Dishonorable discharge. In most cases they will send

you to the stockade for six months or four months and tack it onto your tour of duty.

Mr. X: That's terrible. It kind of destroys all my plans. I had this whole thing worked out, with a mop and bucket, like in "Anchors Away."

Mr. H: I didn't see it.

Mr. X: I think it was Abbott and Costello. It all looks very hopeless to me. (Mr. X tries to show that he is not awed by Mr. H's story of success in military service, although Mr. S had been impressed by it.)

Mr. H: Did you say you didn't have to go in the service?

Mr. X: I said I didn't want to. There is a difference.

Mr. S: I noticed before when you put out your cigarette, you knocked out all of your ashes. Do you always do that?

Mr. X: Yes.

Mr. S: I find myself trying to stop that.

Mr. X: On the subway it happens often that I sit there and if you look and just look out of the corners of your eyes and see your hands, and they look so pink, I don't know, just out of the corner of your eye, they'll be laying in your lap and then if you look down at them, you look at your hands sometimes just laying in your lap, and they look so dead.

Mr. S: I do that. I look at the veins.

Mr. H: I remember reading once that you don't do anything unless you visualize it, and I always wondered, do I visualize my hands moving or do I just move?

Mr. S: The doctor might know.

Mr. P: What would a blind person do in that case, if he had to visualize it?

Mr. S: You visualize in your mind. Blind people visualize a lot of things.

Mr. X: I know a teacher; he talked about visualizing things. He just bought a color TV set. (Attempts to make a *reductio ad absurdum* of the talk by the others. Tries to maintain his superior "cool" attitude. Part of this is his desire to impress the therapist.)

Mr. H: I also read blind people, when they get sight back

they want their blindness back because it wasn't what they visualized.

MR. X: I read a cool story in the *Reader's Digest* in 1958 where a man was blind and he got his sight back, and, like, the first time he ate scrambled eggs, he never saw scrambled eggs before—people just told you they were yellow, which means nothing to you.

MR. H: It must be interesting, the visualization, because they wouldn't have colors. I guess to experience it, one would have to be blind.

MR. X: One step removed from that is being completely objective to view things. Lots of times when I think of the ludicracy and idiocy of being human, I think about purely objective things; about what happens. Like they were building this tract of houses in Pennsylvania and then stopped because, I don't know, they found a fifty-year-old graveyard, a hundred-year-old graveyard, under the tract of land, and all these bones were there and they didn't want to build houses there. And can you feature explaining how these hundred-year-old bones stopped the building of these houses to someone who is, like, from Mars? You know, some being who doesn't know death and who comes from Mars. Even simpler things are more ridiculous. Music is great. Can you picture trying to explain why some people go "ga ga" over square dancing? (Mr. X has many depressive features. The onset of his severe behavior disorder occurred when he was fifteen years old, following the death of his father. His father had been an invalid for a year before dying of cancer of the colon.)

MR. S: I saw a cartoon of a Martian observing the earth and all the stuff we did, cures for medicine, and how far advanced we are, and saying, "But I can't understand why they made striped toothpaste."

MR. X: But there it is, there is a terrible seriousness in all this terrible humor and I see all the ugly humor and it comes up and makes me sick and I say, Why go on? It's a drag.

MR. H: What's the alternative?

MR. X: I know I don't want to die. I can picture myself

sitting down with a bottle of iodine and mixing this up in a glass of chocolate milk to kill the taste, or in a "Yoo Hoo."

DOCTOR: In a what?

MR. X: In a "Yoo Hoo." It's a chocolate drink they make. It's noncarbonated. It has artificial chocolate, artificial milk, artificial water; it's a prime target for me. I can feature making this whole portion and, you know, mixing it up, but I couldn't feature drinking it.

MR. S: You must have hated life.

MR. X: Why use the past tense? There are some days I feel like this and some days I feel good.

MR. S: On those days you hate life, do you go into school with a chip on your shoulder?

MR. X: No, I went into school today and studied like a champ. No, I function very well in my hate gear. I just put it into hate and I function fine. I worry a lot, but I function well.

DOCTOR: Mr. S, your father called today. (This intervention was made to interrupt Mr. X's depressive ruminations and to inform Mr. S of his father's call early enough in the group session that some discussion would be possible before the end of the session.)

MR. S: What did he want?

DOCTOR: What did he want?

MR. S: Yes.

DOCTOR: Well, he wanted to know what best to do about your asking him to have lunch with you. He said that you had said something about going to school and not working. And I told him, don't make up your mind today.

MR. S: Yes. Well, I already mentioned that I thought it would be good to get a part-time job over at his office and pay for my schooling like that.

MR. X: Is this a private conversation? (Mr. X objects to the attention paid another patient. Mr. H follows Mr. X's lead. The subject has been changed, however.)

DOCTOR: No.

MR. H: Yes, that's what *I* was wondering.

DOCTOR: No, go ahead.

Mr. X: You want to work in your father's office?

Mr. S: I sort of pictured that I could work there and pay for my schooling.

Mr. X: That's not getting out very far, working for your father.

Mr. S: It doesn't have to be in his office. I could get a job through him. He doesn't want me to work in another place.

Mr. X: Why don't you get it through you?

Mr. S: Because I saw a lot of girls walking around, going into every door, door after door, and getting refusals. And I said to myself, that will never be me.

Mr. H: I can't agree with you completely.

Mr. X: I didn't say I was thinking anything. I just asked him a question.

Mr. H: Will this be your first job?

Mr. S: No. I had jobs the last four or five years. I have been working, but I never want to bring myself in without anybody knowing me, or just to go in and say I want a job.

Mr. X: You figure they'll say you're not good enough?

Mr. S: No, I figured I'll be like the rest of the people. I felt they were lower than me; they had to go around begging different offices for a job.

Doctor: Why do you laugh, Mr. H? (Mr. H had laughed while Mr. S was speaking. It was important that this communication be brought into the group discussion and clarified. It resulted in fruitful discussion.)

Mr. H: The striking similarities.

Mr. X: They're all over the place.

Mr. H: Yes. Well, I tell myself it's you, but I have the same attitude you have. All of these people down here have similarities. But also, doctor, there are people like me having the same problems. I thought getting overseas, and things like that, this is just me, but it isn't that way.

Mr. X: Can I say something? Quote "normal" unquote people have the same problems, a whole lot of the same problems that we have in this room here. It's not the problems. It's what you do with them.

MR. S: Do you know that for a fact?

MR. X: Yes, I know that for a fact.

MR. S: Is that true?

DOCTOR: Well, what do you think?

MR. X: Sure, it's true. Do you think it's true?

MR. S: Yes.

MR. H: Why not? I mean, everybody has problems.

MR. N. I don't think it's true.

MR. S: I don't think it's a hundred percent true.

MR. X: Don't you think people are nervous when they go out for new jobs?

MR. N: I don't think it's pleasant to walk around knocking on doors. I don't think it's a problem. It's not necessarily a problem.

MR. X: That in itself is not a problem, but the reason we're here is because the same problems everyone else has and has overcome or not even noticed are noticed by us and are large obstacles and out of proportion to us.

MR. H: And then again you can rationalize and say you're trying to meet your problems more efficiently and better than other people do.

DOCTOR: What do you think, Mr. B?

MR. B: I have been listening because I have a lot of problems that have been coming up here. I don't see where I'm too different, not too different at all.

DOCTOR: Mr. S, you asked the question.

MR. S: What question?

DOCTOR: Whether the problems here were like other people have. (The question of similarities of the patients' problems is brought back to the patient who originated it. Frequently the questions asked by patients provoke answers in the patients asking them. Patients do not often ask rhetorical questions, but something similar frequently occurs.)

MR. S: Yes. Well, I thought so in a few cases, but I wouldn't say in all the cases.

(Active discussion continues without much intervention by the therapist. Reading verbatim transcriptions sometimes requires effort although the session depicted may have been stimulating.)

DOCTOR: Mr. P, what do you think?

MR. P: I think the problems superficially are alike, but that our nervousness tends to make them very different. And it's as though we had two strikes against us before we even come to the problem, whereas someone else is going into this problem with no strikes against them at all.

MR. X: It's the same problem.

MR. P: Same problem.

MR. X: Same situation.

MR. P: Before we even get to them we have the certain nervousness, anxiety.

MR. X: Fear.

MR. P: Fear. I prefer anxiety.

MR. X: I don't like the word.

MR. N: There is a good deal of difference between situations and problems. You said a situation might be superficially the same, but you turn it into something else. Other people don't turn these things into problems. The situation, whether pleasant or unpleasant, remains.

MR. H: Were you going to say something to me? I thought you were.

MR. B: Yes, I was. You mentioned London. You were in the service in Europe?

MR. H: Yes. I was stationed in England, in Liverpool.

MR. B: Really?

MR. H: Have you been there?

MR. B: Yes, I visited a cousin there while I was on leave. I was stationed in Germany in the service, you know. What's the idea, you like it there and you want to get back?

MR. S: Did you like it there?

MR. B: I enjoyed myself, sure.

MR. H: Right.

MR. S: Would you like to go back? Did you ever think you would like to go back and live in Europe?

MR. B: No, not to live.

MR. S: Mostly everyone in here did. You did.

MR. X: I have never been there.

MR. S: But you wanted to go to Europe, right?

Mr. X: Yes, I did.

Mr. S: Did you?

Mr. P: I want to go to Stockholm and get the prize.

Mr. S: Did you want to go to Europe?

Mr. N: No.

Mr. X: He's lying.

Mr. N: I don't want to go to Europe.

Mr. X: His secret ambition is to rebuild Rome.

Mr. N: I would much rather be an American architect in America. (Mr. N avoids adjectives or other expressions of his feelings about himself. He fantasies himself being another great architect, perhaps a Michaelangelo or a Leonardo da Vinci.)

Mr. X: I want to be an ugly American. I think that's what I was cut out to be.

Mr. H: A what?

Mr. X: An ugly American. A boorish tourist.

Mr. H: Are you referring in terms of the book?

Mr. X: No, I was referring in terms of real ugly, unwashed, unshaved, uncouth American.

Mr. H: There was the "Ugly American," and the "Ugly American" wasn't ugly in the sense you mean. He was the good guy.

Mr. X: I want to be beautiful, but I call it ugly to be protective.

Mr. H: Why do you want to be ugly, a slob?

Mr. X: If I were a slob I'd feel all the things heaped on me I deserve, and I don't have to say, gee, I don't deserve this, this is what I deserve, and there you are.

Mr. S: If you were ugly, you'd still say to yourself, I'm still a human being and it doesn't matter what I look like.

Mr. X: I'm ludicrous. I don't know, did you ever take a good look at yourself in the mirror?

Mr. H: Yes; I'm a handsome one.

Mr. X: I don't know.

Mr. N: Did you ever take a good look at the "David"?

Mr. X: Who?

Mr. N: At the "David."

Mr. X: Who is "David"?

Mr. N: Mikie's David.

Mr. X: Oh, the statue. Yes, that's ugly.

Mr. H: Is there anything that's pretty?

Mr. X: A whole lot of things.

Mr. S: What's that?

Mr. X: A statue. It's misinterpreted.

Mr. N: By who?

Mr. X: By Mike.

Mr. N: He did a bad job?

Mr. X: No, he misinterpreted the Bible.

Mr. N: Whether he misinterpreted the Bible has nothing to do with it.

Mr. X: I think it's ugly. I think people with horns are ugly.

Doctor: Does "David" have horns?

Mr. N: No.

Mr. X: Isn't that "David," man? Oh, that's "Moses."

Mr. H: He doesn't have horns either.

Mr. X: Sure "Moses" has horns.

Doctor: "Moses" has horns, yes.

Mr. X: Trying to tell me "Moses" doesn't have horns.

Mr. N: How about "The Dying Slave"?

Mr. X: I don't know that one. I think there is a lot of beauty, a lot of beautiful people, but it all makes me very unhappy.

Mr. H: You're really intriguing.

Mr. X: That's why I'm speaking, to intrigue you all, I think. (Mr. X knows that some of his attitudes toward people, although successful in accomplishing his purpose, are based on insecurity and the desire to manipulate other people to a position of use to him. He would rather feel comfortable with people without acting a role.)

Mr. H: You sound so bitter.

Mr. X: It's not bitter. Don't get me wrong. I guess there is a lot of bitterness in it, sure. (Mr. X wants to be understood and helped.)

Mr. H: I must say, you're a wonderful storyteller. Last week you were talking about those wires.

Mr. X: I was just going to tell you a story. Have we time for one more story?

MR. H: I was going to ask, those wires, did you cut them?

MR. X: No. When you ask me about beautiful things—

DOCTOR: Mr. H, how about next Monday at ten forty-five, is that feasible?

MR. H: Not at lunch?

DOCTOR: It's a bank holiday, isn't it?

MR. H: Oh, sorry.

DOCTOR: I'll see you a quarter of eleven on Monday.

MR. H: Right.

MR. X: Is it over yet?

DOCTOR: No.

MR. X: Oh, there is more?

DOCTOR: We're waiting for the story.

MR. X: They asked me about beautiful things. I once met this girl in St. Louis. I had just come into St. Louis. Me and two of these other guys I was travelling with went to this club. In the middle of this club there was this chick with blond hair wearing black leotards. She was a waitress, and I thought "oooooh"—can you write that?—like this is the most beautiful thing in the world. She took me home with her and we come to the house, a gigantic mansion with no furniture, and in the middle of the mansion there was a living room with a fireplace and in the middle of the living room there was a mattress. She sits me down on the mattress and says, Wait a minute, I'll be right back, and runs upstairs. When she comes down, her hair is hanging so nice, just curled down over her shoulders. And she's got this big box and carries it over, a cardboard tomato box, and puts it on the floor and sits down next to me, and it's full of photographs, and she says, Let's look at the photographs. And I sat there with this chick for like six hours looking at photographs of her aunts and uncles she saw last Thanksgiving, her grandparents, her family; like the whole conglomeration of seventeen family albums all chucked into this box. And this is what I mean, you could look at it like a symbolic-type story, you know, because although it happened, it has so much meaning for me. I see this as a realization of things. I had this beautiful blond chick, man, you know, and what did it turn into? Just a farce.

(This story expresses the promise and futility Mr. X feels about many things. This statement was left open for discussion by other members of the group. If the therapist had intervened, Mr. X's isolation and his positive attitude toward the therapist would have been reinforced at the expense of his learning to work with other members of the group.)

Mr. S: Did you end up with anything?

Mr. X: What do you mean, anything? If you mean sex, say sex.

Mr. S: Yes.

Mr. X: No, man, I cut out when the sun came up.

Mr. S: Why did you leave?

Mr. X: It was a drag. The whole thing was a shock to me, a very emotional thing.

Mr. S: Did you try? All the time you were looking at the pictures, going along with her, agreeing with her, you know, this is nice and this—

Mr. X: Well, I didn't push her. I don't push any girl.

Mr. S: But how could I tell my friends I looked at pictures all night?

Mr. X: You don't know my friends.

Mr. H: This happens.

Mr. X: We had a very funny relationship. We were very, very straight with each other, I guess out of defense; if I lie to him, maybe he'll lie to me.

Mr. S: I would tell the truth too, but I would try everything possible.

Mr. X: If you're like the pseudointellectual beatnik, traveling-cross-the-country-car type, it turns into humor and it becomes a bit, a story you can tell at some future time, like now. At the time it meant defeat.

Mr. H: It is humorous.

Mr. X: It's funny. But at the time it was a crushing blow. Like those four fateful words: Are you in yet? That's an old joke. You know, so it's a very crushing thing. I had a series of crushing things. Well, of course, most people wouldn't find themselves in this situation, right? To meet such odd and crushing people. You know, it just happened to be the thing that you walk in and see this beautiful thing. I wanted to possess it. It's like reaching out for an apple and picking up a rotten tomato.

Mr. S: I couldn't understand how you even got her to take you home at first. (Mr. S looks at the literal pleasure-getting aspect of the story. He missed the point.)

Mr. X: Oh, I sat down and I wrote something. We were going cross country reading poetry and literature at different places, at colleges, and so forth, in bars and street corners, and I sat down and started writing this here, and I wrote, Once I saw a swan in a great pool of tar—I don't remember exactly—every time it moved more its feathers became blacker, and I would have saved its life had I not been afraid to dirty my shoes; you know, which is funny; but again, it had serious meaning to me. They showed it to her and I spoke to her and said, Where do you live? and she said, Around the corner, wait till three o'clock and we'll go home. And I cacked out right there and I said "woo hoo," and I couldn't wait.

Mr. H: Where did you learn all these expressions?

Mr. X: "Woo hoo"?

Mr. H: Cacked out.

Mr. X: All over Greenwich Village; Chicago, the south side, Houston, Texas is a good place.

Mr. H: Did you go to all these places?

Mr. X: Yes, I took a trip. We started out to go to the West Coast, but we turned in Houston to Mexico and came back.

Mr. H: Your home is in New York?

Mr. X: New York; Brooklyn.

Mr. H: Do you like the Village?

Mr. X: No, it disturbed me. (Here he begins to look at his acting-out behavior. Mr. X was close to panic at the time he began his peregrinations.)

Mr. H: You said you don't see why anyone can go "ga ga" over square dancing. I can't go "ga ga" over the Village.

Mr. X: I find the Village a terribly complex thing most people don't see living closely together. I lived there for awhile.

Mr. S: I always wanted to live there.

Doctor: Mr. P, what about eleven-thirty on Tuesday? (Appointments for individual sessions were frequently made as casually as this without interrupting the group discussions.)

MR. P: All right.

MR. S: They seem to be people that would accept whatever you are.

MR. N: How did you come to live there in the first place?

MR. X: I went down there when I was thirteen to a bar to hear some jazz, and I met two guys there, songwriters. I went with a friend of mine from high school and he had been there twice before and he had met one of them before. We were just standing around the bar talking and one of them struck me immediately as being a personable and very nice fellow. I became friendly with them and through them met other people who weren't quite so nice, who were more dangerous and more destructively exciting. And after I hung around awhile, when it was a particular time for me to run away, I ran to the Village. But they're not friendly there. The people I met weren't friendly because they had to be very careful. They were involved in many illegal, immoral things which could get them into trouble. They, right? *I* was in it. And after awhile you get very careful of who you say what to, right? So you become cool. That word is fantastic, because in the particular group I was in—I guess you could call it a society—cool meant careful. (Mr. X is referring to his running away and his panicky state following his father's death.)

MR. S: That would be a saying.

MR. X: But there is a difference. People say, He's cool and collected; it means relaxed. This meant careful.

MR. S: Well, you could adapt words to different things.

MR. X: Yes. We had a great many words that were just used by us so just we could use them. Everyone does, bridge players do, chess players do.

MR. S: That was always the thing. I always wanted to live there. It seemed like with them there would be no bullshit involved. If you wanted to get laid, you just got laid, and there was nothing there. None of their other girlfriends would say, Look what she did.

MR. X: Leave us remember there are a lot of guys who

realize the same thing. There aren't that many chicks around. NYU is close by and those fellows can change into dungarees faster than you can light a cigarette.

MR. N: Change into what? (Mr. N's failure to understand "dungarees" appeared to be a part of a superficial defensive trick of not appearing to understand things he knew well. He assumed that most of his immediate knowledge came from his family and social background. He was ashamed of his background. Therefore, anything familiar to him might be contemptible, and to act as if he knew these things might expose him to contempt.)

MR. X: Dungarees.

MR. N: What?

MR. X: Dungarees, blue jeans.

DOCTOR: Well, we have to stop.

* * *

Although the transcript of this session suggests that the communications occurred mainly between only two or three of the patients, all members of the group participated, some on a non-verbal basis. If boredom or negative feelings had become evident on the part of those not doing so much of the talking, the therapist would have intervened.

The therapist's interventions were minimal. He began by introducing the new member. The talk then was taken up by the patients. Mr. P described his interests and ambitions. Mr. H followed with a presentation of his ambivalent attitudes toward work and self-advancement. The therapist intervened a few times to support and protect Mr. H when he was pushed and challenged by the others. Later the therapist asked opinions of several of the patients to allow them the opportunity to participate in the discussion. Appointments for individual sessions were made during this group session for two of the patients.

Chapter 6

THE PATIENT'S FIRST GROUP SESSION

The new patient at his first group psychotherapy session is afraid and curious. The other patients in the group may be annoyed at the disruption caused by the introduction of a new member. Sometimes they are relieved when the arrival of a new patient interrupts a tension-provoking discussion. Inevitably curiosity is aroused. The transference aspects of the introduction of a new member to a group are added to these reactions and dealt with, mostly implicitly, in the interactions in the group.

The new patient may be greeted as a long-lost brother, a missing father, a sought-after mother, an unwelcome sibling, a punitive parent, or other transference figure. The patient's reactions to greetings on this basis can be revealing. The comments of the other patients in the group on such greetings can be useful both to the new patient and to the old group members.

The group is not ordinarily told that a new patient is coming. Announcing the intention of bringing in a new member at a subsequent session does not further the treatment work of the group. Sufficient material is produced when the new patient actually arrives. Another hazard of announcing the expected arrival of a new patient is the possibility that he may not appear.

Prior to attending the first group session, the new patient may ask whether he has to talk. He is told he may be silent if he wishes. The patient who is talkative at the first group session and who is allowed to completely expose himself is not likely to return. It is a part of the therapist's job to intervene when this seems likely.

The patient has been told in advance that the group is composed of patients who have problems similar to or related to his own. The fit of a patient for a particular group is something that is judged as much on an intuitive basis derived from experience and training in group psychotherapy as it is on the statistical and diagnostic characteristics of the patient. Ordinarily the patient will be placed in a group while he is still having individual sessions. An early indication of his fitting into the group is given when he feels he belongs in the group well enough to inquire whether he needs to continue his individual sessions.

A patient who is ignored by the other members of the treatment group from the very beginning often is not suited to the group and should be considered for another kind of treatment. New patients for group psychotherapy have been advised that the group treatment at the beginning is on a trial basis, but the trial should continue over a period of several visits. At times the patient who is at first ignored later develops a rapport with the group that makes it possible for his treatment to progress.

At the first group meeting, several members of the group may be invited to tell the new patient how the group works and what it does. This gives the patients who have been in the group an opportunity to evaluate their own feelings about group psychotherapy and to reorient themselves as to its aims and methods.

Like the patient who is overtalkative, the new patient who becomes overly friendly with one or more members of the group is hazarding a disruption in treatment for himself and perhaps for others. The new patient has been advised during the first group session that social encounters of group members are discouraged and to be discussed in subsequent group meetings. This admonition may be forgotten when anxiety or a desire for immediate resolution of social and other problems becomes paramount in the patient's mind.

At the end of the first session, a new member is usually pleasantly surprised and his anxiety is somewhat relieved. He has found that others who have or have had somewhat similar difficulties have been relieved of some of their discomfort. They have learned ways of living more effectively, even when their problems continue. The new patient's curiosity will have been somewhat satisfied. He looks forward to learning more about himself. He wants to resolve some of his problems and to learn techniques for dealing with problem situations from other members of the group.

At times, a patient with a personality disorder who comes to his first group psychotherapy session learns that other people have problems very much like his own. On the other hand, sometimes the new patient only sees the other patients as sick. He finds they have things about them they think of as "sick" and undesirable that he has about him but he thinks are all right. He learns to question what has been ego syntonic. The shock of putting himself in this category is more than he can bear. He finds the situation intolerable and refuses to return to group psychotherapy. Sometimes he leaves psychotherapy altogether.

This denial of illness is not acted out very frequently, but it does occur. If the patient is seen for an individual session following his first group session, the negative reactions that he has for the group can be taken up and utilized in his treatment. It is generally recognized, however, that patients who utilize denial to a great extent are difficult to treat. By the same token, group psychotherapy is an effective means of treating patients who utilize denial to the point where individual treatment is almost impossible.

For instance, Miss M, a twenty-six-year-old clerical worker in a bank, had become so fearful and nauseous when she attempted to ride the subway trains to and from work that she had been unable to continue her employment. She came from a family whose interests were restricted to immediate day-to-day problems. Their stereotyped and ritualistic religious practices played an important part in their lives.

Miss M had never had an easy time socially. She dated rarely and there were only three or four other young women she could call friends. She had come for psychiatric consultation on the advice of the physician at her office. Her services, which were highly specialized and which she efficiently performed, were so highly valued by her employer that her salary was continued during the time she was unable to work. Special arrangements had been made for her to get the treatment she so obviously needed. If she had been left on her own, she probably would not have come to a psychiatrist.

She had been seen for three individual psychotherapy sessions prior to being placed in a psychotherapy group. A lack of personality equipment and social mechanisms, as the expression of her rigid, constricted personality structure, indicated the need for the kind of help she could get from group psychotherapy.

At her first group session, she was quiet, curious, and afraid. Mrs. E, who is described elsewhere, responded to Miss M's predicament by going into a gory recital of her own murderous feelings toward her infant children and her general hostility and suspiciousness toward almost everyone she knew.

Following this group session, Miss M called the therapist, saying that she was convinced that she had nothing in common with the other people in the group because they were all married and she was not and that, besides, "That woman talked about doing such horrible things." She felt that she certainly would not belong in a group with such a person. The therapist told Miss M that she did have things in common with the other patients, not all of whom are married, and that she should return to the group and tell Mrs. E of her reaction to Mrs. E's lurid recital. Miss M said, "All right, doctor, if you think this is the best thing for me to do," and returned to the group at the next session.

At the next session, Miss M described her reactions to the previous group session. The therapist took this around to several other members of the group asking, "What do you think has been going on here?" Miss H, a thirty-year-old spinster, a remitted paranoid schizophrenic, intelligent executive secretary, replied that she felt "Miss M really wanted to avoid coming for treatment at all, and this had given her an opportunity to overlook the sickness that she actually had."

Miss S, a twenty-nine-year-old single schoolteacher who had been treated for a compulsive personality disorder for four years in individual and group psychotherapy, proceeded to tell Miss M that she too had a fear of traveling on subway trains. At this point, Miss M came back with the statement that she had discovered during her psychotherapy sessions that what made her afraid and nauseous was not the traveling on the trains themselves but the crowds she had encountered.

Mrs. E's response to this discussion was to act surprised and listen attentively.

After the group had discussed Miss M's relationship to it, the therapist pointed out that Mrs. E had on previous occasions used her obsessional ideas of drastic assaultive behavior to shock other members in the group. This brought up the question of the reason for her talk in the group about these ideas. Mrs. E then reported that she had recently become excessively religious in practice, even though she had begun to have doubts about the existence of God because she had been having so much trouble.

The day following this session Mrs. E called the therapist to say she wondered whether she should return to the group since she had felt so uncomfortable. She complained that the therapist had been letting her make a fool of herself by not calling her attention to her using her obsessional ideation to shock other people, although she said she had previously thought of this possibility. This transference acting out of Mrs. E was one of many manifestations of her extreme ambivalence.

She was reassured that she should return to the group and continue her treatment. She did this.

Actually, the therapist should have called her attention to the incident without saying he had noticed it before.

Chapter 7

THE TASKS OF THE GROUP PSYCHOTHERAPIST

The group psychotherapist has the primary responsibility for maintaining the group as a therapeutic entity. He does this by selecting patients for group psychotherapy, orienting them to this kind of treatment, and helping them to carry out their part of the therapeutic work in the group.

The second major task of the group psychotherapist is to make the group effective as a therapeutic modality. He does this by arresting disruptive moves of patients and stimulating meaningful interaction within the group.

Like other communications from the patients, seductive overtures directed at the therapist or other members of the group have to be recognized and dealt with for what they are. Often, such overtures are responded to before they are recognized. Bearing this in mind, the group psychotherapist should constantly be prepared to interpret sexual, social, and politically seductive material. He should refer most of the seductive behavior to the group by asking such questions as, "What do you think ＿＿＿ is doing now?" or "What do you think ＿＿＿ is really interested in?" or "How does this sound to you?" in a respectful, yet questioning manner.

This means of polling the group is a useful technique in maintaining both the level of interaction and the discussion of any issue that comes up. When the patients are ready to drop an issue, they should be permitted to do so. This will become apparent after the first or second patient polled on an issue changes the topic or gives an irrelevant answer. At this point, the therapist should stop his intervention and allow the group talk to take its own course.

Provocative behavior will, at times, require a direct prohibition by the conductor of the group. He may say to a patient engaging in behavior that is obnoxious by general social standards that it cannot be permitted. At times, if a patient is upset and unable to behave properly, he may be asked to leave and return at another time when he feels better.

Assaultive behavior can be precipitated by the therapist or the group. This should be prevented by the verbal interventions of the therapist. A part of his work with the group consists of his intervening to convert a discussion from a provocative to an interpretive aim. At times, he must stop discussion of an inflammatory topic and initiate discussion of something less provocative.

When behavior occurs that is sexually seductive or physically assaultive, it may mean that the therapist, in some way, has incited the patient unwittingly. Self-inspection and self-appraisal are constantly necessary for the group psychotherapist. If he becomes aware of a negative feeling toward a patient or a sexual response to a patient, he must be extremely cautious. The relationships between a therapist's negative feeling toward a patient and the patient's destructive and self-destructive behavior are well known. This risk is particularly important in treating patients whose backgrounds are different from that of the therapist.

From his self-appraisal, the group psychotherapist can at times better understand a patient or a group. If he finds that he is awfully tired with a certain group, he should wonder what he is so tired of. He may even ask the group why they think he feels so tired. If the group psychotherapist feels angry at the group or a group member, even knowing that he has an irrational anger and the cause for it, he may say to the group, "I am in an irascible mood today. I don't know why," or some such comment. It is important to say such things because groups of patients are often more aware of the moods of the therapist than individual patients because group psychotherapy demands more activity of the therapist.

It is important that the internal problems of the therapist be handled in such a way that the therapy can progress. If the therapist finds that he feels angry and the cause is not immediately apparent, he may, by reviewing in his mind the immediate discussion in the group, find the cause in some subtle assault from one or several patients. He may use his appropriate response to bring out the negative feelings of group members. Once these are exposed, it is then possible to work with them in furthering the therapeutic work of the group.

There should be very little reason at any time for patients in group psychotherapy to be realistically angry at the therapist. If through some oversight he is constantly late or does something else that might be annoying to the group, he should consider first the reasons for it, then apologize to the group, and change his behavior if he can. If he finds that he cannot modify his behavior he should think of doing some other kind of work.

Groups are constantly changing. Some of the change occurs as new group members come into the group and old patients leave. New patients must be added to replace those who improve and are discharged, those who come only infrequently, and those who drop out. A high rate of patient turnover in a group raises questions about the group psychotherapist, except in situations where external circumstances cause this to happen. An example might be a group in a receiving hospital where most patients would be seen only for a short period of time.

Groups in which there is almost no turnover of patients raise other questions about the group psychotherapist. Ideally, as patients improve and need to come less frequently or not at all, new patients are added to fill the vacant places in the group.

Perhaps the most important aspect of the therapist's interventions in the group psychotherapy is the timing of his interpretations. A group psychotherapist who determines in advance what he is going to say at a group meeting is, in effect, planning a lecture or perhaps a sermon to his group. While lectures and sermons have their place, the psychotherapy group cannot really be considered an audience or a congregation. The group must be followed by the therapist or conductor with interventions as subtle and unobtrusive as possible. His guidance should be keyed to cues picked up from the group. *Non-sequiturs* should be confined to announcements of a change in time or place, or other necessary announcements about the physical arrangements for the next meeting or a change in the schedule.

While the conductor of the group must pick up and call attention to the important themes, he must do so unobtrusively, else the patients will feel pushed and will leave. The handling of the resistances must be handled with discretion. It is important that a distinction be made between resistances to treatment and real impediments to group psychotherapy.

The aim of the treatment in group psychotherapy, as in any psychotherapy, is to influence favorably the functioning of the patient. This does not mean simple symptom removal, because to remove a symptom and thereby claim a cure would be like shooting down an enemy's flagpole from a distance and thereby claiming the fort had been conquered.

The relation of the elimination of symptoms to the work of the treatment is fairly complicated. Many patients with personality disorders complain only of chronic mild depressive symptoms that are expressed as chronic dissatisfaction, fatigue, and irritability. Patients who have obsessions, including the obsessional aspects of delusions and hallucinations, will probably never be entirely free from these symptoms. It is possible, however, that treatment will add enough new material to their total store of mental operations and ideas that the obsessional ideas will be matched, countered, and sometimes inundated by other material.

In some patients, inappropriate ideation can be treated by the reductio ad absurdum that can occur in the talk of group psychotherapy. This kind of exaggeration and isolation of atypical ideation puts it in its place and reveals it as awkward and unessential for the patient.

The general aim of group psychotherapy is to help patients function more effectively and more comfortably. A patient who is unable to work, or able to work only with a great deal of tension, should be expected to work or to work more efficiently with less emotional strain. Patients who have difficulty in interpersonal relations should learn in the group ways of getting along with other people that enable them to enjoy their social contacts with less anxiety.

The role of insight in the cure is to provide a rationalization to the patient for altered and improved behavior. Technical terms should be avoided in the treatment. The insights, the new understandings the patients learn should be in the ordinary language used in the group.

The use of technical language and scientific terms to describe human behavior can easily convert a psychotherapy group into a class in psychiatry or an indoctrination. The patient does not come to be given a course in psychiatry or to be indoctrinated into a system of thinking. He comes to treatment for help with his problems. This help should have a rational scientific basis; however, the science of the treatment is the problem of the therapist and should not be foisted onto the patient.

Psychiatrists who do a consultation practice often see patients who have had the experience of being treated by "therapists" who appear to have only read some books, then set themselves forth as counselors, advisors, or persons with other designations that imply help with emotional and interpersonal problems. These patients speak at times a veritable flood of pseudoscientific language that is meaningless. It appears that they have learned to speak new words and thereby have avoided facing problems in living. They have avoided the opportunities for realistic solutions. Their would-be-therapists have ignored the realities of emotional life by operating a distraction composed of pseudointellectual verbal formulations isolated from everyday problems.

The better functioning of the individual is the best criterion of meaningful change. An improvement in functioning does not always require an elimination of the presenting symptoms nor does it coincide with the development of psychological mindedness. The presenting symptom may remain. A phobia or an obsession that brings a patient to psychotherapy may continue, but one would expect the symptoms to be less troublesome at the conclusion of a successful treatment.

Delusions are probably never given up. A patient may become aware of some of the factors in his background and his psychological makeup that shed light on his delusions, but the delusions themselves cannot really be expected to disappear. Other material is put into the adaptional systems of the individual through his experiences in group psychotherapy that lessen the importance of delusional thinking and orient the patient toward more realistic overt behavior.

The determinants for the behavior of a patient, including his mental activities, can only be added to. The factors that give rise to delusional thinking can be combined with other determinants to neutralize them. If this occurs to the point where the patient can be relatively free from disability, although the discomfort is not completely alleviated, he can be said to have been treated successfully.

The group almost automatically provides the consensus of opinion in its microsociety and thereby influences the systems of adaptation that form an important part of the ego of each patient. The therapist's role is to further this work by providing some consistency, the other philosophic criterion of reality. He keeps the discussion open-ended and avoids coming to rigid conclusions and definite closure. The discussion involves the interpretations of internal and external reality. This enables a continuing consensus to persist.

While it is vital that the conductor of a group be able to be unobtrusive in his interventions, he must also be able to take a strong stand in a very explicit way at times. He must be able to intervene directly to prohibit a patient from becoming disruptive if that becomes necessary. The therapist must be able to intervene directly invite a shy or mute patient to participate, at the same time avoiding upsetting him.

In contrast to patients who must be supported in their attempts to avoid distressing situations, other patients require direct support in their efforts to be active socially, sometimes sexually, in business, and in other ways. The therapist must give approval and support to patients in these endeavors unequivocally.

Parenthetically, it must be noted that to certain patients encouragement is interpreted as a demand on the part of the therapist. This can lead to a self-defeating kind of destructive and self-destructive acting out. For this reason, support and encouragement must be delivered in a way that leaves the patient freedom of movement and avoids compulsion.

Ordinarily, to serve this purpose, interventions of the group psychotherapist should be limited to those in which he prevents a patient from being hurt in the group and to those required to keep the group discussion going.

Miss C, a remitted catatonic schizophrenic woman, required protection by the therapist when other members of the group pressed her with questions about her social and sexual life. She had been exposed to a variety of sexual approaches from her disturbed alcoholic brother on occasions when he would return home at night drunk. She can be said to have resorted to a catatonic stupor to escape this troublesome stimulation. Her response to almost any provoking or exciting stimulus was to become, as she put it, "numb" and to "have trouble walking" because her legs would become "stiff." When the talk in the group sessions concerned dating and marriage, Miss C would become visibly upset when she was drawn into the discussion. At this point, the therapist intervened to say, "Miss C is better to remain single and not date. There is no requirement that everybody date, that everybody be married, or, for that matter, that everybody be sexually active. I think it may be better for you to avoid these things, Miss C, because they may be too much and too upsetting for you." The expression of relief on her face was immediate.

Again, timing is vitally important. The therapist would not start a group session by saying before any discussion had begun, "Miss C, you should not be active sexually," nor would the session start with, "Mr. A, you should be more aggressive in your social life." The time for intervention is when the topic has been broached.

For instance, the intervention to support Miss C's avoidance of sexual stimulation was made following her telling the story of a disagreeable situation with a strange dentist. Mr. A had been asked by another patient in the group about his social life before the therapist had intervened to encourage his activity.

A patient who monopolizes the talk in the group has to be stopped. The group psychotherapist intervenes directly to do this. He says to the monopolist, "Let's see what the others think about this, Mr. N," and then proceeds to ask Mr. O what he thinks.

Mr. O may say that he was not listening and thinking of something else, whereupon he is asked to talk about something else if he wants to do so. Sometimes he does. If Mr. O does not desire to speak, then Mr. P or Mr. Q may be polled in the same way. If none of the patients wish to talk, the therapist may be obliged to discuss the material the monopolist has been presenting. This predicament does not arise often, however, if the therapist has been aware of his feelings and reactions to the group and to the monopolist and by this self-awareness avoids intervening on account of his own context rather than responding to his knowledge of the group.

The therapist's reactions in this kind of situation can inhibit the talk of the group and provoke silence. With very disturbed patients, silences should be allowed to occur, providing they are of brief duration. The therapist should not hesitate to interrupt a silence to ask questions or to present his own views. Repeated episodes of prolonged silence indicate the need for self-appraisal or supervisory consultation for the group therapist.

In a group in a public hospital clinic containing many chronically incapacitated patients of low social and economic status as well as bright college students, Mr. N described at length his difficulties in getting and keeping jobs. He described his failure to pass a test to be a Western Union messenger. He told the group how he had been fired after working a few hours in a grocery store where he had failed to put the cans on the shelves properly, how he failed to operate the cash register properly at the checkout counter, and how he had ultimately failed at sweeping the floor.

This chronically incapacitated patient had the appearance of a healthy young man. He remarked that his brother, who was confined to a wheelchair, could get a job and was working, when he could not. When Mr. N described how physically incapacitated his brother had been, the therapist raised the question as to whether the brother were worse off than Mr. N. The other patients took this up, pointing out that Mr. N might be more disabled than his brother. Another point made by another patient was that the disability of Mr. N's brother was evident to everyone around, whereas mental disabilities are not immediately obvious.

The other members of the group took this up, discussing the difficulties they had due to having a record of hospitalization for mental illness or of psychiatric treatment. They discussed the way in which most people will try to help a person who is obviously physically disabled, whereas when a not-so-evident mental disability becomes known, people generally are likely to shy away from the patient.

The role of the therapist in raising meaningful questions is illustrated here by his comparing the disabilities of Mr. N with those of his brother. This question had to be raised in a way that would avoid hurting Mr. N but would not avoid the reality of his mental illness.

Mr. T, a nineteen-year-old Negro high school dropout, psychologically and intellectually unsophisticated, was in the same group. He had been referred to the clinic by his probation officer. He had been arrested for assault and attempted rape. He denied all illness, yet came regularly to the group sessions. He participated little verbally, but paid close attention to discussions of the problems of other patients in becoming adults and the discussions that the other men in the group had about their relationships with their mothers, wives, and girlfriends.

Mr. T's behavior at home had improved since attending the group. Mr. N, who was verbally aggressive, asked Mr. T what was wrong with him, whereupon Mr. T looked appealingly to the therapist who made no answer but waited until another patient in the group began to talk. If Mr. N had pressed his question, the therapist would have intervened to protect Mr. T, who had no real understanding of his predicament. His benefits from the treatment were derived from the general setting and the total group atmosphere. To have pressed him about specific thoughts and feelings would have hazarded his disintegration.

It is well known that the group psychotherapist does not always answer questions or respond verbally to talk directed at him. What is not so apparent is the opposite kind of activity, the seemingly gratuitous intervention of the group psychotherapist who, for example, interrupts a discussion to ask a patient not active in the talk a question about a new topic he knows the patient is likely to talk about.

The purpose of this kind of intervention is to cut off further discussion of the previous topic to avoid a definite conclusion or closure of the discussion. Only a few of the many determinants for a problem can be taken up at a time. Consequently, it is important to prevent a patient from concluding he has found the cause for the problem prematurely.

Once a patient feels he has reached an intellectual conclusion about something he is likely to think of it as finished business and not want to think again about the factors determining an aspect of his behavior, even though his feelings have not been relieved nor his behavior changed.

After an emotional reaction has been modified and function improved, it is often easier to look back and talk about some of the determinants that were implicated in a painful conflict.

Once a change for the better has occurred there is no pressure for a definite conclusion about a symptom. If the patient can function better more comfortably, then the formulation he proposes may have some relevance to the change. Most of the time these formulations have only tangential application. The changes observed have developed during the course of the open-ended discussions of some emotionally charged material.

Mrs. Ch came to group psychotherapy for several months trying to get some pat formula or drug to explain or relieve her chronic depressive reaction. Only after she began talking about her current life situation did she begin to improve.

She was chronically depressed. She lived with her mother whose permission she sought for almost every act. When she described her home life, it sounded like a tyranny to the other patients. They remarked about this. Mrs. Ch then for the first time told of her childhood with a semi-prostitute mother (now living a quiet life), who placed her daughter, the patient, with one relative, another relative, and institutions in between, during her stormy early life.

Her disastrous marriage at age sixteen had been an effort to escape. The fourteen-year-old daughter of this marriage now receives her mother's constant devotion and attention.

When these elements were brought out in the group, Mrs. Ch began to improve. She began to be more realistic in her relationship with her mother and daughter.

If a group conclusion had been permitted in the previous discussions in which Mrs. Ch complained about her worthless husband, the treatment would have been effectively hindered. When the new material emerged, there was no need to intervene to prevent closure. Since they had been tempted previously to come to conclusions on insufficient data, the group was now reluctant to do more than explore and exclaim at the new revelations. The treatment could continue.

It was only after the therapist had intervened directly to ask how Mrs. Ch spent her time that the relationship with her mother was described.

Another reason for seemingly somewhat abrupt intervention by the therapist to change the subject is to maintain the discussion of the group at an active level. When a topic has been talked about to the point where the interest of the group is no longer engaged, the therapist may intervene to introduce a new topic.

The tasks of the group therapist are work, self-discipline, and self-deprivation. His rewards are increasing knowledge, the satisfaction of carrying out a technique with proficiency, and the fees and salaries received.

Chapter 8

THE WORK OF THE GROUP

The task of the patients in the group is to learn more about themselves and other people. This learning occurs as each patient talks about himself, his ways of running his life, and his ideas about others. From this talk, he gets an understanding of how he appears to himself. How the others see him becomes apparent to him from what the other patients say.

Each patient brings to the group the system of mental devices he finds useful in meeting his internal needs in his own society. This system of internal mechanisms and social devices originates in the impressions he receives from the matrix of his primary social group. In our society, this is usually the family. The *modus operandi* of each individual is therefore determined, to a large extent, by social factors.

At times, the style of behavior will be a reaction against rather than a positive result of the primary social influences. The biologically determined inclination to imitate and learn by example is at times not possible as the result of an abnormality of the central nervous system. At other times, the immediate environment provides adverse reactions because of its own extremes.

Family pressure, which determines the personality organization, is succeeded by social pressure as the individual grows up and leaves the family for a great part of the day. The learning that takes place as the result of social pressure is refined in individual and group psychotherapy to influence the patient favorably. The intact functions of those with defects of the central nervous system can be utilized to develop a more efficient set of social responses. Ideally, patients should have biologically intact equipment; however, stigmata of heredity or environmental damage are frequently encountered.

In group psychotherapy, each patient speaks what he feels able to say. It is impossible for a patient to free-associate in a group setting. Of necessity, the deliberate verbal productions represent personality organization. The aspects of personality that are emphasized are recognized for what they are by the patients. The group psychotherapist will understand the latent meanings of these productions in the group setting. By protesting too much about certain attitudes and by omitting others, each patient paints a portrait of overly vivid hues and strikingly blank canvas. These productions make patterns that are usually intelligible to the group and almost always to the therapist.

The therapist's interventions should be carefully timed to avoid interfering with the work of the group. His job is to facilitate its work. Most of the interventions, no matter how directive, should be unobtrusive. A useful technique for this purpose is to raise questions rather than to make directive interdictions.

For each man in the group, the other members, both men and women, can give him their opinions and thereby knowledge of the many things a man can do, think, and feel. The same applies to each woman in the group. In this way, the deficient aspects of each patient's personality development can be pointed out and alternate modes of behavior can be suggested.

The group represents a larger sampling with a greater diversity of personality types than the family or other social group that each individual usually has as his determining social matrix. A person brought up in a family where parents were overly repressive can learn from the consensus of the larger microsociety of the group that inhibited behavior is not the only approved kind of reaction in social relations. Likewise, the individual who has been seduced by his family into exaggerated assertiveness and hyperactivity can similarly learn the areas in which this form of extreme behavior is inappropriate.

As is well known, patients often are able to see in other people defects that they have themselves, and this ultimately becomes exposed in the work of the group.

One of the philosophic criteria of reality, the consensus of opinion, can be approached in group discussions. In a properly run group, consenses are being approached constantly. This does not mean that ultimate answers or final conclusions have to be reached in the group setting. The fluctuating continuity of reality is implicitly recognized in the consenses of the group, provided the discussions are kept open-ended.

Miss S constantly quizzed other patients in the group as to their feelings about almost every topic and freely expressed her opinion about the appropriateness, good taste, and fashion of almost every bit of behavior described. Eventually, another woman in the group pointed this out to her. She took it up in the terms that Miss S must be very insecure and fear that she would be an odd person or left out. This was suggested by her great concern about the styles and roles of conformity.

It was further pointed out to Miss S that she never talked about anything bothering her. The question was raised as to what her reason was for coming to treatment. Of course, it had become evident that her overconcern about being acceptable had revealed difficulties in getting along with herself and other people. In this way, the self-portrait each patient paints by overemphasizing certain colors and outlines calls attention to its blank areas.

The total consensus of reality, including the individual intrapsychic reality, is thus alluded to and taken up in each group session.

Another patient, Mr. H, a twenty-two-year-old emotionally unstable, single, white laborer was constantly getting himself into trouble by impulsive behavior. Most recently he had become angry because the interviewer at an employment service to which he had gone to collect his unemployment compensation had asked him to provide a list of places where he had tried to find work. He had spoken in a loud voice, complaining that he was being mistreated and in the presence of the interviewer had torn up the registration book in which he was required to record his visits and payments.

When he came to the group therapy session that evening, he spent several minutes complaining loudly of how stupid he had been to mess himself up in that way, yet at the same time he complained equally loudly about the excessive demands of the interviewer and the employment service.

Because of his erratic behavior Mr. H had been unable to

complete high school and had not been able to hold a job longer than eight months. He described these disappointing experiences during his lamentations.

To everyone's surprise, Mr. F, a thirty-five-year-old single elementary schoolteacher who had come to treatment for help with his effeminate attitudes, agreed with Mr. H and supported him in his complaints about the government and its regulations and family inquiries about how he ran his life. This aspect of Mr. F's personality had not been brought out before.

Mr. I, another teacher, had come to treatment for relief of his overwhelming fears of having such diseases as cancer and heart trouble. A borderline obsessive-compulsive, he was married and the father of three children, successful at his job, and very active in community and local political organizations. Mr. I expressed surprise at Mr. F's revelations. He pointed out to both Mr. F and Mr. H that their feelings were unrealistically excessive.

Mr. W, a single, white college graduate and a remitted paranoid schizophrenic, had earned his living at times as a fencing instructor. He carefully, politely inquired of Mr. F and Mr. H, concerning the details in the reality of the incidents in which they both complained about the curiosity and interest of their relatives in their lives.

In these interactions, the excessive, overt antagonism and complaining of Mr. F and Mr. H were abraded by the excessively conformist attitudes of Mr. I. The friction of these conflicting views served to even out the attitudes of these three, and Mr. W's clarifying inquiries emphasized the reality for everybody in the group.

In another case, Mrs. E, who has been mentioned previously, during her third year of treatment had described in detail the arguments she had with her husband. In discussing the incidents with other members of the group, she became aware of the excessive anger she felt toward her husband during their arguments over little things. She said at one point, "I feel like I have to have him make something up to me," although she was not aware of what it might be. She became very annoyed at Mrs. T, who spoke of her own past feelings of antagonism and resentment toward her husband, which were not in keeping with the realities of the problems in their relationship.

When most of the group agreed that Mrs. E's anger and resentment toward her husband were inappropriate, she accused the people in the group, including the therapist, of criticizing her unduly and being unfair to her. During these interchanges, Mrs. T told Mrs. E that she herself had stayed in the hospital longer than necessary after a suicidal attempt because she had been afraid she could not carry out her duties as a wife and mother.

These exchanges between Mrs. E and Mrs. T in a group of women illustrated a part of the "identity committee" effect of a psychotherapy group. To enhance this effect, the therapist picked up Mrs. E's comment about feeling that her husband had to make something up to her and asked several members of the group what their reaction was to this comment, having in mind, of course, the problems of masculine-feminine attributes and their expression in the work that women do as compared with the role of the men in their lives.

Mrs. E's progress in treatment was marked by her recognition that her feeling that her husband had "to make something up" to her was inappropriate to her actual experiences with him. She then began to question her other attitudes. Questions from other members of the psychotherapy group in which she was treated had spurred her own questioning of herself.

Mrs. T's fears about doing her job as a wife and mother were handled in the same way and yielded productive discussion. The discussion of Mrs. E's and Mrs. T's feelings about masculinity and femininity tended to increase the inventory of ideas and devices for interpersonal relationships of each of the women in this group. In a group that includes both men and women, the same kind of discussion of masculinity-femininity can be more sharply delineated by culling the opinions from the men concerning their expectations of women and by inviting the women to speak of their ideas about what women should provide for men and vice versa.

Mr. X had been in psychotherapy for six years for treatment of a severe personality pattern disorder with depressive, paranoid, and homosexual elements. In a group of young men he described a dream concerning a homosexual relationship with a rich friend who had loaned him a large sum of money the preceding evening.

Mr. X had had no homosexual relationships for over five years, had married, had returned to college, and had decided to borrow money to go on to graduate school. Four months previous to this session, his wife had given birth to their first child, a son.

Mr. M, who has been described previously and who had been in this group for three months, suggested that this dream might have something to do with Mr. X's feeling toward his rich friend as a father. This in turn led to a discussion of Mr. X's role as a husband and father. Each man in this group of young men was drawn into the discussion of how they felt about growing up and becoming husbands and fathers. Again, each patient's stock of mental sets concerning his masculine-feminine feelings about himself, the other members of the *present micro*society generally was explored and presented to the *group*.

One aspect of the supportive function of the group is illustrated by the patient who said in a group session, "Here everybody has a problem and nobody's going to make fun of you."

These examples show a vitally important working aspect of the psychotherapy group and how it adds to the mental capital stock and the inventory of social maneuvers available to each patient in the group.

In this reality-oriented therapy, the internal reality can be approached by a careful examination of the external reality.

The following excerpts of actual group sessions illustrate the work of the group.

Chapter 9

VERBATIM EXCERPTS FROM DISCUSSIONS OF OTHER GROUPS

The following verbatim excerpts of group psychotherapy discussions are a partial record of group sessions conducted by a psychiatrist in his own office as part of his private practice. Most of the patients who participated in them had been under treatment for several months.

The excerpts are representative of the verbal exchange that take place in group psychotherapy discussions. They are given to illustrate the function of the group psychotherapist for teaching purposes.

These verbatim excerpts happen to be of groups containing all women and all men. This selection of patients was done from patients available for group psychotherapy at the time the verbatime records were used. They illustrate the incidents of actual group psychotherapy sessions and are representative only. It would take several volumes of verbatim excerpts to illustrate all the points described in the text.

A GROUP OF WOMEN

The group was composed of six women, most of whom were in their twenties and thirties, married, and mothers. It included a spinster stenographer, Miss H, who was about forty years old. Miss C has been mentioned before.

DOCTOR: How are you, Miss C?

MISS C: All right. My father is doing much better. They let him get out of bed now for an hour or so. Doctor said that he'd like him to start walking around a little bit. The only thing he complains about is his legs. He says they're like rubber. But

---

These excerpts are taken from Stenotype transcripts obtained as described in "The Use of Recorded Minutes in Group Psychotherapy: The Development of a 'Readback' Technique." (*op. cit.*)

doctor said that has a lot to do with that he was in the bed so long that he's a little weak. (Miss C rarely spoke of herself. She viewed life in terms of her parents and her relationship with them. Her treatment was primarily supportive.)

DOCTOR: Uh-huh.

MISS C: I got to the hospital a little late yesterday and I had told my mother that I would be there late, and as I was going in I seen my brother and sister-in-law and I didn't realize it was them until I was up a little bit closer. But then, I don't know, I hesitated and I said no, I wouldn't do that, and I just walked past them, and that was all there was to it. I mean, I didn't get too much like I did the other times. (Miss C's difficulties with her brother have been described previously.)

(Mrs. G enters the room)

DOCTOR: I guess I better get out another chair or two.

(Doctor puts out chairs)

DOCTOR: How does that sound to you, Mrs. N?

MRS. N: I wasn't thinking about it. I don't have anything to comment on it.

(Doorbell rings)

MRS. E: I didn't hear your last remark. You said you walked past your brother?

MISS C: Yes.

(Miss H enters the room)

MRS. E: And what?

MISS C: I just walked past my brother and I just kept walking. Usually, I get very upset and I find great difficulty trying to control myself. But last night I didn't find that. I could just walk by and I didn't feel bad or anything about it, just like they were strangers, I didn't know them. It didn't bother me walking by them. (Miss C reports that she has handled her troublesome feelings toward her brother by avoiding him. In doing so she indicates she is seeking support and approval. No comment is made, the inference being that silence means consent or, in this case, approval.)

DOCTOR: Miss H, how are you?

MISS H: Fine, thank you.

DOCTOR: Do the capsules help?

MISS H: Oh, yes, quite a lot.

DOCTOR: Good. You're taking two capsules twice a day? (Medications are discussed openly in the group.)

MISS H: Yes, sir.

MRS. N: My husband called this afternoon and he's really quite annoyed with me; no sleeping, nervousness, tension. He says that something has to be done. I feel terrible.

MRS. E: What seems to be bothering you?

MRS. N: I'm extremely nervous, extremely tense, and I'm not sleeping well.

MRS. E: Do you know what you're nervous about? (Mrs. E has improved. She has developed some psychological mindedness and begun to recognize some of her inappropriate emotional reactions.)

MRS. N: No. I'm afraid. I have peculiar fears, and they're not—they don't make sense. They really don't. Because they are the same fears I came into group therapy with, and all of a sudden the fears recur. And they're right there; they're not gone. I've gotten along better for longer periods of time, but now I am quite upset. (Mrs. N is a chronic paranoid schizophrenic. She hallucinates frequently. She has managed to do a creditable job of housewife and mother to her husband and two sons. Her treatment has been supportive and in the service of encouraging repression. Some interpretive statements have been useful to her at times. She uses the group to help her find a consensus for reality.)

MRS. G: What fears do you have?

MRS. N: Well, for example, if I go to sleep, if I go to bed earlier than my husband and he will come over to say good-night to me, if he hovers over me, he terrifies me. It's terrifying to me. This is something that is very upsetting to me. It makes me feel terribly afraid. I don't think this is the first thing; this is not the first reason. The feelings must be within me to begin with, so that any action will frighten me.

MRS. G: When you say you don't sleep, how much sleep do you get? Do you have absolutely sleepless nights?

MRS. N: No, not completely. I would say that I have about four hours of very light sleep, the dozing sleep, where it's a sleep where I'm listening. My younger child has had a temperature, he hasn't been too well, and I have been listening. But I don't think that was the main thing. I find again that music soothes; it's very relaxing. I put on the earphones and that helps a lot. But I realize that I'm afraid, and I'm afraid in the daytime too, and there is no reason for the fear.

MRS. E: I felt afraid at times too. I can't understand why. I don't know, it seems silly to me.

MRS. N: Oh, I know that they're strongly sexual, there is a very big conflict and it's a very difficult thing for me to understand or recognize.

MRS. G: Do you take tranquilizers at all? (Mrs. G changes the subject to tranquilizers when sex is mentioned. Mrs. G, a severe obsessive-compulsive with depressive episodes, has tried to avoid sexual problems. She constantly denied any psychodynamic cause for her troubles, yet was never late for a psychotherapy session and rarely was absent.)

MRS. N: Oh, yes, yes. Usually I have the Deprol, and then when I get more uncomfortable it's Thorazine, and then something to sleep. I'm just a collection of little pills. They're so pretty, at least.

MRS. E: Do you talk to your husband about all these fears?

MRS. N: Yes. And the doctor says I talk too much to him. I've tried talking to him and he is a very understanding person, but there is still a point where it's so personal that I don't think an explanation can be accepted or—can be accepted by him. I mean, he understands that I need to be here, because there have been many times when I felt very confident and felt that I could get along without it. He's the one who says you can't because he knows, well, he's going to suffer if I don't have the group and the medication. But I am disturbed. I'm disturbed because the feelings are so physical, the tension is so physical. And it's not just taut nerves.

MRS. G: I get so scared with everyday living, sometimes my heart pounds.

MRS. N: No, I don't get that way. I don't have that.

MRS. G: It's not palpitation or anything like that. It's just plain fear.

MRS. N: Yes.

MRS. G: And they're silly fears, just as you say that yours are silly, that you can't—you're still afraid, recognizing that there is no basis for them.

MRS. N: Well, there is a basis and the basis is that I slept in my parents' room until I was eleven years old, and so that there is a very strong, bad background. And certainly I was aware, and so the fear upon hearing their sexual relations or being frightened at their arguing, which I would hear as a very young child, and then having my father come over to me to explain, and I would nearly always be turned towards the other side, so that this action on the part of my husband is one that upsets me terribly. It just takes me back very quickly. It's something that I can't seem to get away from. But the thing is, why does this happen only at certain times? Why not all the time?

MRS. G: Or better yet, never.

MRS. N: Right, never. It's gotten so sometimes when I call him on the phone he even sounds like my father when he answers the phone. I find this very annoying.

MRS. E: When I was in the hospital, one of the doctors told me that when you become emotionally sick, you regress into childhood, or something like that. Maybe that could explain the fears. I mean, you know, children have fears.

MRS. N: Yes. I'm responding the way I did when I was a small child. I'm an adult now, but the response at that time is one which is many, many years old. I don't think I'm regressing. I'm acting the way I did then. In other words, that's not gone from me; that fear isn't gone. I don't have any security that has taken the place of fear, because it's almost—it's a fear of injury.

MRS. E: Is that what you're afraid of?

MRS. N: Yes. I'm sure it's a fear of injury. I think so.

MRS. E: How are your sexual relations with your husband?

MRS. N: They're good at times. At times they're not good.

MRS. E: Are you afraid of injury then?

MRS. N: No. I think they're fairly normal in the respect that relations can be very satisfactory to me at certain times, when I'm relaxed, when I'm comfortable, when I'm most receptive. And other times if I'm overtired, tense, or whatever it is, then I'm not going to be as satisfied, but I understand that too. I think that's like anything, anything you do.

MRS. E: My sex life hasn't been too good lately. I don't know, I just can't be bothered. It's a funny feeling. For awhile I was enjoying sexual relations but now I just can't be bothered. And I don't know what it is. I'm so absorbed in myself, I have no desire for anything. And I always resent when my husband comes near me. And I don't understand it. (Mrs. E. recognizes some of her reactions are unnecessary and inappropriate.)

MRS. N: Is he attentive to you in other ways essentially?

MRS. E: I think so, but he needs a lot of sex, my husband, and I don't need quite so much. And sometimes I resent it a little bit. But I don't know, we're having all kinds of troubles now. I have to see the obstetrician on Monday, but I'm still bleeding and my husband doesn't want to come near me. So he says as long as I'm taking these pills and I might get pregnant, he doesn't think I should have a baby while I'm taking pills. And since I'm Catholic and I can't use contraceptives, no sex life at all. So I don't know what to do. (Mrs. E's husband had neurotic difficulties that interlocked with those of his wife. He was phobic. Her defensive-aggressive approach would anger him at times, whereupon she would become more aggressive and bitter conflict between the two of them would occur.)

MRS. M: You can't use contraceptives? What was all the talk about deciding whether to have a baby or not if—

MRS. E: Well, I've been using the rhythm method and it's worked for me. But it's not enough for him.

MRS. N: I heard something interesting today. I was speaking to a friend; she's pregnant and her sister-in-law is pregnant, and both have been given Dexadrine by their obstetricians.

MRS. E: What's that?

MRS. N: It's a diet pill. I thought that was very strange,

because I know that did terrible things to me not pregnant. I mean, I just couldn't imagine taking this while pregnant.

MRS. M: What is it?

MRS. N: It's to control appetite and to stimulate, I think, some kind of activity within you.

MRS. M: Burn up your calories.

MRS. G: I think I took Dexadrine for the first few months when I was pregnant. I started off with two pills a day and that hopped me up too much, and they had cut it down to one. But it increased my appetite, rather than decreased it.

MRS. M: Why would you, as slender as you are, take it?

MRS. G: Well, they still don't want you to gain.

MRS. M: I know, because I was very thin. I was underweight and they still didn't want me to gain.

MRS. G: He let me gain twenty-five pounds, which is more than they usually do, but I had a terrible time keeping it down to twenty-five. I didn't take it very long. I just took it for awhile.

MRS. M: Doctor, how would it be—I thought of this little plan during the week; I never put any of my plans into action; maybe if I had I would be better off—if I paid you six dollars a week? I'll tell you what that means, just right now to get started with something, because my share of the bill is three dollars a week and this way I would be catching up. And I got a raise, not merit or anything, but the first of the year everybody gets a few dollars. So is that all right with you? Or what do you think of that? (Mrs. M's transference demands can be seen in this manipulative handling of her fee for treatment. Her procrastination led her to be late in paying her bill, which was almost completely covered by insurance.)

DOCTOR: You mean this would bring your bill up to date?

MRS. M: In four or five months it would bring it up to date and I wouldn't be four or five months behind, let's put it that way. If I started doing this five months ago, we'd be all up to date. Believe me, I've got another problem—I haven't been—I've got something else on my mind right now, but this I did think of, it's the only thing I could think of, the only constructive thought that I had about this situation.

DOCTOR: Your share of the bill as it stands now is three dollars a week?

MRS. M: Yes. If I had been paying you when I caught up in the summertime, if I had paid you every week, I wouldn't have got behind, so I thought maybe I should start paying you each week, because it will be easier to do that than to try to save it or any other method.

DOCTOR: Well, we can try it.

MRS. M: Okay. As I say, that's the only thing I can think of that I can do right now.

DOCTOR: Did I give you a bill, Miss H?

MISS H: Yes, you did.

MRS. N: Something else my husband's commented on. He says that I don't answer questions correctly, that I answer out of context, that I'm speaking on the telephone and certain questions will be asked, I answer in an incorrect fashion. In other words, not what the people are really asking me, as if I don't understand the question they're asking. And the same thing happened this morning. I had a house call; this pediatrician came to see (her child) and I realized we did more talking about our schools and his daughter than my child with a temperature. And it's a little bit distressing to me, because it didn't occur to me until after he had left that his instructions were much too quick and very general. It's true it's a routine thing, but I still realize that I should have asked him more questions and should have stopped him because he was talking too quickly. And I realize that I do this in many situations, so that I don't get the correct information. It makes me feel a little unhappy. (In a sense, Mrs. N can be said to be inviting the therapist to a competition with her husband. Her statement suggests she wants the therapist to be like a good father as compared with her husband, who is critical of her way of using the telephone. She later expressed her awareness of her inappropriate behavior. This ability to recognize her difficulty in mental operations makes her treatment much easier.)

MRS M: Don't you think you're being a little hard on yourself? (Patients in the group support one another very effectively, as is illustrated here.)

MRS. N: No.

MRS. M: Do you think she is?

MRS. E: I think so.

MRS. M: A little demanding too much of yourself? After all, if you had gotten some point confused in your mind, you could have called him in his office. Of course, he wouldn't have liked that; that would have been inconsiderate.

MRS. N: No, it took me twelve hours to get in touch with him yesterday.

MRS. M: I don't mean to come back to the house.

MRS. N: I couldn't even get in touch with him for six hours to even speak to a resident. All I got was messages. My husband said people who are on welfare get to see a doctor and here we're paying, we're not charity patients, and we can't get one.

MRS. M: I thought pediatricians made it a point to be talked to.

MRS. N: Yes, between eight and nine in the morning. If that time passes, there are places, either in the hospital or finally there are office hours, but to give you information to tell you about a house call, it's a very intricate—it seems ridiculous. I don't understand it. It's the strangest thing. I mean, I know certain hours have to be kept, but this is—

MRS. M: Why don't you switch to another pediatrician if this one was so difficult to get?

MRS. N: This man we called is the one that was recommended to be called in an emergency, because our regular pediatrician did not have hours and I couldn't bring (her son) down in a taxi, take him to her office. And then the person who might have made the house call was not available, so I cancelled the call. Then I called this other person who I had been told to call and that was in the evening, and then he finally made the appointment for the morning and he did arrive and it was fine, I was very glad, and he got there in the middle of the morning, which was marvelous. I didn't expect that much. But you know, these are very—they can be important. They can be. They can be in situations where the child might be really very ill and then I wouldn't know how to press the issue to make it seem, you know, this is important, this child should be examined; it's this type of a thing.

(The hostile transference reaction expressed in these comments about doctors is mostly resolved by members of the psychotherapy group. In individual psychotherapy such hostile reactions could disrupt treatment.)

Mrs. M: Well, in that case, in a real emergency, what you're supposed to do is get in a taxi, if you have to call your husband, and take him to a hospital. I know it's easy to say. I always know what everybody else should do.

Mrs. N: We've done it. My husband once had to take _____, in fact, it was a hospital, I don't know, to the outpatient area, and then it took about half an hour until a nurse came to find out what was wrong with the child because there was no one around, and then when the doctor finally did come around to see (the child) it was quite awhile. It's a very, very slow situation and there weren't that many people there. You know, it's strange. And fortunately, the children aren't sick often, and even when they are, when they have been sick, it hasn't been anything terribly serious, for which I'm glad; because, believe me, I think I'd get pretty wild.

Mrs. G: How high a temperature was he running?

Mrs. N: It hadn't been a high temperature. It had been between a hundred and a hundred-two for several days. This is not a high temperature. But I was told by the pediatrician last winter that there was a possibility of something peculiar happening to him at this funny in-between temperature and to watch out for it and let her know, and I remembered this and I became preoccupied, nothing extreme, but the amount of time that it lasted, he did need some kind of medicine besides aspirin, which we wouldn't be able to get without a prescription.

Miss C: My mother received an invitation to a baby shower and they included me in the invitation and this is from—it's my—I guess he'd be maybe a third cousin to me; it's his wife's niece, and I really don't know her. I mean, I've met her once or twice, but I haven't been to the wedding and I don't know her. I just know her by sight and I told my mother I wasn't going.

So my mother said, "I probably won't go either but I'll send a gift." And I said I probably wouldn't send a gift because I don't know her that well and I wasn't to the wedding and I think the whole thing is ridiculous to invite me to the shower. So she got upset by this. And, I don't know, she started reciting different lines, something about a bird, no matter how high he flies, you have to come back to the earth for water, and you can't go around knocking everybody down. I don't know. She started like that and I just turned around and said, "good-night, Mom," and I went to bed, and I don't think my mother likes what I'm doing, but I just think it's kind of silly to go to a shower that—I don't know, I just don't have any interest in going. And I thought it was quite odd that they would invite me.

DOCTOR: I think you were right, Miss C. (Supports Miss C in her expressions of hostility as avoidance.)

MRS. E: Doctor, I've been feeling pretty comfortable this week and I'm still taking medicine. Do I have to take it when I feel all right?

DOCTOR: Well, maybe you can begin to cut it down some.

MRS. E: You mean just cut out one pill?

DOCTOR: Well, you might try cutting out the one in the morning and see what happens.

MRS. N: Oh, there was something else. Last Friday night I went to the movies and I think I called and talked to you about this, and I was sitting in the movies, my husband had a person sitting next to him, so he handed me the umbrella to hold, and I was on the aisle seat. I was sitting holding this umbrella, and I felt so resentful and so angry at having to sit there. This is unreasoning. I felt like taking it and driving it right into the ground. I really did.

MRS. G: Were you mad at him for making you hold it?

MRS. N: Yes. Yes. Just take it and smash it. I never carry one. I'd rather get wet. I wear a raincoat or a coat with a hood; I will not carry one. (Mrs. N's anger is based on some irrational, probably symbolic, meaning of the umbrella or her holding it for her husband.)

Doctor: Listen, are you still trying to lose weight?

Mrs. N: Of course.

Doctor: Stop it, please. Period. Do you understand me? It's not good for you. (This direct advice is the kind of statement that is required at times.)

Mrs. N: I'm not taking anything.

Doctor: I know that.

Mrs. N: I eat well.

Doctor: Well, maybe.

Mrs. N: I do.

Mrs. E: I wish I could lose a few pounds. Since I started taking the medicine, I've been gaining by leaps and bounds. I don't know, I've been trying to cut down on my food, but that's no good. But I don't think—it's terrible. I've put on about seventeen pounds. I was too thin before, but now, I don't want to get too fat.

Doctor: What do you want to lose so much weight for?

Mrs. N: I want to be skinny.

Doctor: And then?

Mrs. N: I want to be a skeleton with some flesh on it, with nothing that anyone will want to grab. I guess that's as clearly as I can put it. (Thinking of her flesh as something to be grabbed by another person is part of Mrs. N's thinking related to her identity problems. Her ambivalence about being caressed and being fondled is expressed in this statement.)

Mrs. G: It's not such fun being so skinny.

Mrs. E: It isn't.

Mrs. N: It's not so much fun being fat either.

Mrs. G: But you're not fat.

Mrs. N: All right. I want to be thinner. I really do.

Doctor: Please stop the diet. Or I could put it another way and say, why don't you stop worrying so much about food? It's upsetting you.

Mrs. N: Food?

Doctor: Uh-huh. It's what you diet about, isn't it? You don't have to gain weight, but certainly it's not good for you to diet; right now, anyway, or to try to lose weight.

MRS. N: I don't think I should wait any longer. I don't think I should wait until my late thirties or early forties to try to diet.

DOCTOR: Well, I don't know when to wait for, but I tell you as your doctor, it's not good for you now. It's not good for your head, you know. (The direct advice is presented again.)

MRS. N: Yeah; uh-huh. The brain that doesn't work?

DOCTOR: Well, it works. Why don't we hear what happened last time, part of it anyway.

(A tape recording from the preceding session is played.)

MRS. N: I talk a lot. (Mrs. N's reaction to hearing the tape recording. The following exchanges show how the various patients react to the recording and to one another.)

DOCTOR: Do you think she talks a lot, Miss H?

MISS H: Not too awfully much, I don't think.

DOCTOR: Mrs. E, do you think she talks a lot?

MRS. E: No, I don't think so, not excessively.

DOCTOR: Why do you think she would say that, Mrs. G?

MRS. G: Well, I think she does talk a lot. I don't find it objectionable in the least. I envy her.

MRS. N: No, I hadn't realized that I had interrupted you last week.

MRS. G: I hadn't realized that you had either. When?

MRS. N: Oh, talking about food and cooking.

MRS. E: I have realized something—well, I've said it before—how much my son looks like my mother-in-law; he's the image of her, and sometimes when I happen to look at him I see the same expressions on his face that I see on hers, and it disturbs me. I don't like it at all. I don't know. It's not that I don't get along with my mother-in-law, but I just don't like her very much. And I don't like my son to look like her. I mean, every time I look at him it reminds me of her, you know. Maybe that's why I had these mean feelings towards him; I don't know.

MRS. N: But didn't you have the mean feelings towards him before? I mean, if the baby is like her, not only looks like her physically, but if she takes care of him, certainly he is going to imitate a lot from her. Didn't you have mean feelings about him before you got sick?

MRS. E: I was sick before I had him. I was sick three years ago. And—oh, no, I didn't have these feelings until he was about nine months old.

MRS. G: My little girl looks just like my mother-in-law, whom I don't like particularly.

MRS. E: Does it bother you?

MRS. G: No, it doesn't. Neither of my children looks anything like me at all.

MRS. E: Oh, I don't want him to look like me, or anything like that. But it does bother me.

MRS. N: My children are interesting combinations. They are. It's very difficult to say which family is which, you know.

DOCTOR: I think there is something very important in this, about this talk about the children and who they look like. Do you have any ideas about it, Miss C?

MISS C: No.

DOCTOR: Mrs. M?

MRS. M: No, I haven't, but I'm very interested. I'm wondering what you mean.

DOCTOR: I don't know what there is in it, but it seems to be something that's important to maybe you, certainly Mrs. G, Mrs. N, Mrs. E.

MRS. N: I want my children to be nice looking, attractive looking children.

MRS. E: I want my son to be the same way, but I feel he's not. I don't think he's nice looking. I can't help it; it's the way I feel. It's a terrible way for a mother to feel about her own child.

MRS. N: Yeah, but what is it that makes a child attractive or appealing?

MRS. G: A good expression?

MRS. N.: Yeah.

MRS. G.: My children are both most attractive. My little girl, and I say she doesn't look like me, so I can brag on it, but she's a little doll. She's a little blond, blue-eyed, almost white-haired child, and she doesn't look like she belongs to me.

MRS. N: Well, I know that when I was a little girl, there was a woman, a friend of my grandmother's who used to come to the house and call me (a girl's name) because she said I look exactly like my father, I didn't look anything like my mother, and I used to resent this terribly. Everyone: "Oh, you look exactly like your father." And this was always a real pain with me. I wanted to look like my mother.

MRS. G: I used to be told I look just like my mother and I used to—

MRS. N: The same.

MRS. G: You're the spitting image of your mother, just like mother, I'd know you anywhere.

MRS. N: It's funny.

(The identity feelings of these women as separate individuals rather than as copies of their mother or father are expressed in terms of their children and at times in terms of their parents.)

MRS. M: Yeah, they used to say the same thing about me and my three aunts and mother, you know, four. But so what? Sometimes I didn't like it, sometimes I did; I don't know.

MRS. E: The doctor told me something one time, he said, "You love the child anyway, no matter what he looks like," so I do love my son; I do. But I do have these feelings about him sometimes and I would love to understand why and just get to the bottom of it.

MRS. N: I did something funny. I know it was funny. (The name), my younger child, has heavy eyebrows, the way I do. They're almost in the exact shape and form. And I pulled out all my eyebrows so I would have skinny eyebrows so that I would be different, so that (he) would be like (himself) and not like me. You know, usually it's a matter of tweezing or shaping because of style or fashion, but this time the reason was different, it was because (his) eyebrows were heavy and mine were too. Another thing, I wouldn't want my children to be overweight. I think this is something that I've been concerned with in myself, my own family; I try to have them have very good eating habits.

(Here her problem of her identity as a distinct, separate individual from her child is expressed. The other patients take this up in the discussion. They provide Mrs. N and the others with a variety of ideas.)

MRS. M: What I would think, with all the unhappiness that you have had with being mentally sick and feeling miserable about it, that you would be more concerned with how they would feel inside than how they would look on the outside.

MRS. N: Oh, I am very concerned.

MRS. M: Well, how can you be so concerned about so many different things so intensely? It's no wonder you're about to collapse.

MRS. N: Well, you've answered it. I mean I'm not about to collapse, but I get upset.

MRS. M: I mean, I'd get exhausted the number of things you're concerned about and all equally intensely. I don't know how you have so much intensity because it's not very logical to look at it that way. Of course, I guess there are hundreds of other things you could be—you're picking out some, it just seems to me that you have so many different things you're concerned about with them, whereas I'd be more concerned about them being happy inside, a little bit carefree, you know, things you're not and wish you had for yourself and for them, I'm sure.

MRS. N: Well, they are as carefree as they can be within safety.

MRS. M: No, I don't mean carefree in action. I mean a light-hearted feeling. I don't say that they don't have it, but—

MRS. N: Oh, boy. They break the place because they're so lighthearted.

MRS. M: I mean how carefree they will be when they're a lot older.

MRS. N: I know.

MRS. M: Because what if one is stocky or one is gangly, but that is so relatively unimportant.

MRS. N: No, I disagree with you, Mrs. M.

MRS. M: I knew you would.

MRS. N: It is terribly important.

MRS. M: It is not.

MRS. N: Particularly to an adolescent. There are feelings of inferiority, feelings of being unacceptable.

MRS. M: It can be overcome much easier than being mentally ill.

MRS. N: Many a mental illness is strongly related to what the image is. (The identity problem is stated directly here. This leads to a worthwhile discussion in which the reality is emphasized.)

MRS. M: No it isn't. A mental illness causes what the image is.

MRS. N: I disagree with you.

MRS. M: Sure, there is a source of unhappiness. A perfectly normal, good-looking person that is crippled in the middle of life suffers from that time on from a feeling of unhappiness over any deformities, but that is not the same thing as saying that causes and is a prime source of great unhappiness.

MRS. N: I know it. I have experienced it.

MRS. M: What? You're deformed?

MRS. N: I have experienced it in myself and I have seen it to a great degree in other people.

MRS. M: Your overweight is not a great deformity.

MRS. N: My own aunt is one of the most difficult personalities but whether overweight is a cause, I don't know, but certainly the two are there and it's a very, very big problem, and this is something that can't be overlooked or pushed aside.

MRS. M: How about the overweight people that are happy and adjusted and how about all the good-looking, medium-sized people that are miserable?

MRS. N: There are bound to be in either one, but you can't deny that overweight and underweight has a very strong influence on how people feel and think.

MRS. M: You're thinking of it as a primary cause, I can tell by the way you're acting.

MRS. N: I don't know what you mean by a primary cause, Mrs. M.

MRS. M: You wouldn't talk about it that way if you didn't feel that it was a primary cause.

MRS. N: I don't know what you mean by a primary cause.

MRS. M: You think if one of your children is overweight or

underweight or stoop-shouldered, it's going to precipitate a very unhappy state necessarily.

MRS. N: No, I don't think so. You're the one who just said it.

DOCTOR: Well, we have to stop.

* * *

The relationship of obesity, dieting, and identity were apparent in this session.

Playing back a tape recording of a preceding session is a variation on the "readback" technique.*

VERBATIM EXCERPTS FROM
THREE CONSECUTIVE SESSIONS OF A MEN'S GROUP
Session 1

At this session the group consisted of eight young men. These excerpts were chosen from the available excerpts of group psychotherapy to illustrate the continuity of the group's interactions. The discontinuous aspects of open group psychotherapy sessions, the changes in the patients of the group due to the absences of group members and the arrival of new patients, can be seen to occur as a minor discontinuity within this series of sessions. One patient in this group, Mr. T, came irregularly. Mr. I was a new patient to the group session.

(Doctor introduces Mr. I to the group.)

DOCTOR: How are you, Mr. E?

MR. E: Fine, thanks.

DOCTOR: What have you been doing?

MR. E: What, today?

DOCTOR: Yes.

MR. E: Looking for a job.

(Mr. T enters the room. Doctor introduces Mr. T to the group.)

MR. E: Sometimes I get the feeling that these epileptic actions, that's what I call them, could be controlled by willpower. (Mr. E had petit mal seizure discharges on EEG. Although he

---

* "The Use of Recorded Minutes in Group Psychotherapy: The Development of a 'Readback' Technique." (*op. cit.*)

These excerpts are also taken from stenotype transcripts obtained as described in "The Use of Recorded Minutes in Group Psychotherapy: The Development of a 'Readback' Technique." (*op. cit.*)

reported occasional very brief lapses of consciousness during the day, these had neither responded to medication nor noticeably interfered with his school or work. Mr. E did not like medication and at times relied on Christian Science.)

DOCTOR: Well, there is one kind of epilepsy in which something like this can be done, but I don't think it generally is true; you don't have that kind. Why? What brings this up?

MR. E: Well, it might be that I just am not—know how to relax, sort of, physiologically or psychologically. (Mr. E utilized several devices in his attempt to deny illness.)

DOCTOR: Have you been having trouble?

MR. E: No, no more than usual.

DOCTOR: How have things been going with you, Mr. J?

MR. J: All right.

DOCTOR: I like your tie. (Mr. J was wearing a tie almost identical to that of the therapist.)

MR. J: Thank you.

DOCTOR: Very similar.

MR. H: Birds of a feather.

DOCTOR: Well, yes; birds of a tie, anyway.

MR. D: Sartorial birds.

DOCTOR: Yes. Mr. H, can you tell Mr. I and Mr. T what we do here?

MR. H: Well, actually we sit pretty much the way you see us doing now and occasionally one of us will speak about something that may be bothering him, and sometimes some of us may join in the discussion and give good, helpful advice, and sometimes it's just helpful to know that someone else may feel the same way. No? (What Mr. H says to the new patient depends in part on his transference reactions to the newcomer and his transference reactions to the therapist. Requesting a patient to tell a newcomer about the work of the group causes the patient to review in his own mind what he thinks has been happening in the group. What he says can be illuminating to the therapist and the old patients as well as the new.)

DOCTOR: Well, if that's your honest opinion, that's the way it is for you.

MR. H: Yeah.

DOCTOR: Do you agree, Mr. D?

MR. D: Certainly do, yes.

DOCTOR: Have you gotten anything out of this kind of treatment?

MR. D: I think so. The realization of much of what will benefit me has to come from me and also a few perspectives of looking at things that I wasn't aware of. There has been a marked improvement, especially last week. I had sexual intercourse.

DOCTOR: Well, we'll give you a gold star. (To emphasize the transference relation implicit in Mr. D's reporting his success to the therapist.

MR. D: A small one because there are other problems to overcome; they'll get bigger as we go along, I guess. But I'd say a marked improvement, in attitude and all.

DOCTOR: As I recall, last week you told us it had been six months—

MR. D: No, about two and a half months. A waning period, but I think my whole outlook has been better.

DOCTOR: How are things with you, Mr. T?

MR. T: I saw my wife tonight and she told me that she would come back to me after she had a chance to think it over; she's going to get her own apartment and think about it. She says in about six months she'll come back, if everything turns out all right. She wants to find out if I'm going to keep working.

DOCTOR: She's put you on probation.

MR. T: Yeah, after she left me.

DOCTOR: What do you think of that, Mr. I?

MR. I: It's quite a story.

DOCTOR: Mr. E, what do you think?

MR. E: I sympathize.

MR. T: With who?

MR. E: With the situation.

MR. T: Well, you don't know the story so I don't see why you say you sympathize.

MR. E: Well something like this, I mean, that appears to have been at least attempted or failed or partially failed is unfortunate, just in terms of the success or failure of a human endeavor that may or may not have merit is difficult to say. But it just creates emotional problems to the people concerned, which might be good in the long run but not for the short term.

MR. I: I was going to ask him, does he really miss his wife?

(Mr. T nods.)

MR. D: How long have you been separated?

MR. T: We're not actually separated.

MR. D: Or living apart.

MR. T: A month.

MR. J: Why did she leave?

MR. T: Because I wasn't working, I guess; because I was tied to my mother's apron strings, let's say, at that time. My mother would call me up and tell me something; I would go along with what she said.

MR. H: How long have you been married?

MR. T: Two years.

MR. J: Do you think your wife was right in what she did?

MR. T: Yes, I think she was right. I would have done the same thing. I've had a chance to think it over. I see it her way. But she won't see it my way.

MR. D: What makes you say that, the fact that she's—

MR. T: She doesn't believe that I'm going to stay on the job, in other words.

MR. D: Have you had many jobs in the two years you've been married?

MR. T: Yeah.

MR. D: What seems to be the trouble? Why do you find difficulty in holding them down?

MR. T: Well, I have epilepsy.

(Mr. A and Mr. L enter the room.)

MR. T: I have epilepsy and I had an attack on the job and stayed out awhile and here my mother comes into the picture again and says don't go to work, you're going to get hurt, and I would listen to her. (Mr. T's seizures were well-controlled when he took his medication.)

MR. D: In other words, it isn't actually your ability to perform.

MR. T: No, no, it's my own fault—I was all clogged up, let's say.

MR. D: Was your wife aware of this when you were going with her?

MR. T: Yeah, sure; I told her. She says now that she wants to think it over, she wants to get her own apartment, be alone.

MR. J: Do you think you can keep a job?

MR. T: Yeah. When I started the job the man told me it would be a two-week trial period. After the first day he gave me regular hours and a regular day off, and everything.

DOCTOR: Are you working now?

MR. T: Yeah.

DOCTOR: What are you doing?

MR. T: A mechanic. See my hands?

MR. D: Is that what you normally do?

MR. T: Yeah. We went to court yesterday; she took me to court, family court, and we would sit in front of this woman and tell her our stories and she would try to get us back together, try to patch it up. But my wife would sit there, she really has a nervous condition, she would sit and bite her nails, tap her foot, cry—

MR. D: It's probably quite an emotional experience for her too.

MR. T: Well, she was that way before this, except I didn't realize it. I just passed it by, but everything built up. And now she's in between her mother and her sister and she can't think for herself. That's what I think. So she says she's getting her own apartment; I don't know if she'll get her own apartment or not. She says she has a job typing at home. Of course she can't go out; she has to take care of the baby.

MR. D: Oh, yeah?

MR. T: Yeah. But she still wants to go through with an annulment and the woman down at the relation court says she has no grounds for an annulment; if she has a baby how can she get an annulment? But she still insists she can get an annulment. This is my first time here, so I don't know what you're thinking.

(Doctor introduces Mr. L and Mr. A to Mr. I and Mr. T.)

MR. T: So then she says to me she doesn't want to live (here) any more; she wants to live in (another borough). That's where she is right now; she's living with her mother. (Mr. T has kept the group interested in his story. Really very little open interaction has occurred although the interest of the group has been maintained.)

DOCTOR: Maybe she'll change her mind.

MR. T: She was crying all the time that I was there today. I think she's just on the verge of coming back. I think she's sick of staying there. About another two weeks and she'll be back.

DOCTOR: What do you think about this, Mr. L?

MR. L: I don't know, I couldn't really hear, you're talking very low. I couldn't really understand; something about your wife found out you had epilepsy now and she left you?

MR. T: No, that has nothing to do with it.

MR. L: Because of something else?

MR. T: Because I wasn't working, that's why she left.

MR. L: How come you weren't working?

MR. T: Because I was on compensation. I got hurt on the previous job that I had and she wanted me to go back to work.

MR. L: How long have you been married?

MR. T: Two years.

MR. L: Probably more than just because you weren't working; there had to be another reason, I guess.

MR. T: Oh, arguments, all kinds of tension, worries.

MR. D: Had you lived close by both parents or with them?

MR. T: No, we have our own apartment. We live on (a street address); they live on (another street).

MR. D: Did they visit you a lot?

MR. T: No, I visited them. I dragged her over to them.

MR. D: I think by and large, I don't know about Mr. H's early marital experience, but I think there comes a time you have to grow away from your parents. (Here some interaction begins. The relations of each man in this group to his mother are reflected in his reactions to Mr. T's story.)

MR. H: Cut the umbilical cord.

MR. T: That's right.

MR. D: I know there came a time with me. It took a little bit of doing. We lived with them; that made it difficult for us.

MR. G: I lived around the corner.

MR. D: That's why I asked if you lived with them.

MR. T: I know now that I was wrong whatever I did.

MR. L: It takes two to have an argument. Maybe she was wrong too in some ways. You can't blame yourself entirely. What sort of condition do you have? Is it frequent? Is it bad?

MR. T: It can happen any time.

MR. L: Do you completely pass out?

MR. T: Yeah. But after every argument I used to have with her I used to have an attack. This time I didn't have one. I think maybe I broke through, or something.

DOCTOR: You may not be taking your medicine regularly. (This is a direct statement of the therapist's opinion. It is utilized to emphasize the reality of the patient's illness.)

MR. T: No, no, because I was on a kick I didn't take the medicine.

MR. A: No connection between the psychological and the attacks?

DOCTOR: Nobody has ever been able to prove it.

MR. T: I'm different.

MR. A: Let's put it this way, every case that I heard, I've heard four since I've been there, it seems every time whenever nervousness occurs, the attacks occur. You can deduce a little bit from it.

DOCTOR: That's pretty hard to prove.

MR. A: What do you mean pretty hard to prove?

DOCTOR: You mean *post hoc propter hoc*, is that correct, Mr. E?

MR. E: Yes.

DOCTOR: If you mean a causal relation, the two things may be caused by something else and there is very good—

MR. A: True, true. I don't doubt that. I'm familiar with the causal theory but it's also generally asserted that if there is constant conjunction occurring, after a certain number of incidents that there are probably necessary facts involved.

DOCTOR: Well, the only connection that I'm willing to buy is that when an episode is coming on that the individual is apt to be more irritable and argumentive; they're emotionally labile.

(Phone rings. When the doctor answers there is no response.)

MR. H: Maybe it was somebody's wife checking.

DOCTOR: Your wife?

MR. T: I don't think so.

DOCTOR: I don't think so. Why would you say somebody's wife—

MR. H: I just thought I'd be funny.

MR. T: He meant your wife.

DOCTOR: My wife?

MR. T: Joke. (This apparently represented an attempt to obtain the therapist's support for the patients who felt threatened by their wives and mothers. The therapist did not play the game because it would serve in the denial of the fears these patients had about getting along with women.)

MR. L: I'm scared. I thought by—how long have I been coming here, about a year?

DOCTOR: Uh-huh.

MR. L: I'm still not better yet at all. I figured by this time I would be. So what is it, a year and a half until I get out of school? If I'm not better then, it worries me. I don't know; I don't seem to be improving. Sometimes I improve and sometimes I go right back to the way I was before.

(Mr. L speaks out despairingly after the discussion of Mr. T's epilepsy and troubles with his wife and mother and the discussion about getting along with women. His mother had treated him with a distant repressive strictness as an infant and small child. The discussion of mothers continues.)

* * *

MR. L: I just feel I could be having a much better time, you know, in whatever I do, if I could just snap out of this.

MR. A: Oh, you know, doctor, I've found one valuable method of handling my mother, and that is, you know, she's nervous sometimes, but you know, she listens sometimes. So what you do is you press her by asking questions. You know, she says, "This is the law." So I say, "Why is that?" Then after awhile—

MR. L: This is annoying, you know.

MR. A: Then after awhile, after two or three questions, you get her to say something completely ridiculous, and then after awhile she bursts into laughter; just maybe two or three questions. It's not that annoying, except when maybe she's in a bad mood; then I won't do it. But the past couple of weeks it's worked a couple of times. I've been able to control her a little by that technique.

MR. D: What does she do otherwise?

MR. A: This is the law.

MR. D: She lays it down to you.

MR. A: Yeah. Then I say, "why?"

MR. L: I usually do that when somebody tells me I should do something. I just don't like to do it if I don't know what I'm doing; when I was little I always was that way too.

MR. A: In these type of moments she's just a little bit irrational.

MR. L: You just expose it to her.

MR. A: Yeah. Not a little bit. I guess, as you say, you expose it to her. But it's worked.

MR. E: Do you think your mother is overconcerned with trivia?

MR. A: Yeah, sure. My mother has got problems of her own. I guess ineradicable psychological problems, and she knows it.

MR. E: And so you invented this game?

MR. A: Well, let's just say that perhaps. But it's necessary perhaps. I mean otherwise it's unbearable at times.

MR. D: She lays the law down to you so often?

MR. A: Yeah. Well, not too much anymore, you know, but what gets me about her is that very, very often she'll be—she'll just refuse to do something on very irrational grounds and, you see, this is what I'm trying to control.

MR. L: I notice I also have a lot of trouble getting girls really to go out with. I've never had that many really. I've had a fairly good amount; not that many really. I figured maybe things have changed. I haven't gone out in awhile before this and I must have gone out about five Friday nights in a row and I don't seem to be getting anywhere at all. And I'm not like I used to be; I can dance now; I'm not afraid to walk up to anyone. I didn't seem to be succeeding. I seem to be comparing everybody to my girl and I only go up to the best ones. I don't see anything wrong with that. I don't seem to be getting anywhere. I'm talking to them for awhile and they say excuse me, and then I run up to another one. Last Friday night I was talking to about seven girls and I didn't get anyone and the two kids I went with each got one.

(Although Mr. A describes difficulty in getting along with his mother and difficulty in getting along with girls he would like to date, he doesn't correlate the two phenomena.)

MR. A: But you had fun trying.

MR. L: I didn't have fun. One of my friends was drunk and he walks up to a girl and starts talking; she didn't walk away from him.

MR. D: Maybe your approach needs polishing.

MR. T: You have to know how to talk to them.

MR. L: What do you consider knowing how to talk to them?

MR. T: Well, you have to know how yourself.

MR. L: That's what I figured.

MR. T: It's your personality.

MR. L: Maybe I got a rotten personality.

MR. A: He didn't say that.

MR. D: Maybe you count yourself out before you start.

MR. A: That's me.

MR. L: I go up, I figure once they start talking I figure I've got one already; we talk and talk and dance.

MR. A: Maybe you talk too much.

MR. L: No, I let them talk as much as they want. I just don't talk about what school do you go to and this and that. I don't do that. I get around to it eventually, but I try to vary it as much as possible. (Mr. L also complains about difficulty in talking to girls.)

MR. A: Let them talk about themselves and flatter their own vanity; that's what they say in the books. As I said, I have no personal experience to verify that.

MR. L: As I say, I walked away too. I didn't seem to be getting anywhere. A lot of my friends said you have to be more aggressive. I don't know, you talk to them for awhile, big deal; I'm not going to throw myself at someone.

MR. D: Why don't you try it once?

MR. L: I tried it. It hasn't been recently though. I just want to know that I could get someone. I enjoy going with the girl I'm going with now.

MR. D: That's what I was going to ask you. Why is it so important?

MR. L: I want to know that I can get someone else too.

MR. T: In other words, you want to play the field; you just don't want to go with one girl. I can give you some numbers.

MR. L: I got a couple of phone numbers last summer. I didn't bother calling them up. It's just the idea that I could get their phone numbers; that seems to be the game I seem to be playing. (Mr. L's inability to have warm relations with girls is expressed in his coolly describing his getting girls' phone numbers as only a game, not the real thing.)

MR. D: You just want to see how many conquests you can make.

DOCTOR: You were going to give him some numbers?

MR. T: A few.

DOCTOR: I don't know whether that would help, frankly. (This represents an exploratory intervention. If the patients had responded with a question, the relationship between getting phone numbers and getting along with women would have been questioned. The fear these patients have of women is handled by avoidance.)

MR. T: I don't use them. I get them from my friends.

DOCTOR: These are not used numbers then.

MR. T: I don't use them. That's what's wrong with me; I stick to one.

MR. D: What makes you say that's what's wrong with you?

MR. T: Well, everybody else says—all my friends say they like to go with other girls.

MR. D: Are they married?

MR. T: No. One of them is, yeah.

MR. D: It makes a little bit of a difference.

MR. T: One's engaged, one's married, one's—

MR. D: Does the married one go with other girls?

MR. T: No.

MR. D: Then it's quite easy for him to tell you to do it.

MR. T: He says it because my wife left.

MR. D: Then it isn't just the idea of going. In other words, it's therapy. Did I say something wrong?

MR. A: No, doctor.

MR. D: Oh, thank you.

MR. H: Have any of you gentlemen ever had this thought? this has occurred to me, somehow it's a frightening thought, this is kind of in line with what you were saying. I looked this up. I see Descartes did a lot of studying about it. I looked it up in a lot of theological books. Have you ever thought why you're you? It's kind of a frightening thought. (The identity problem reappears and is taken up quickly in the group discussion. This continues for a great part of the session. The sexual aspect of this is implicit in its following almost directly the discussion of the relationship of these men to women.)

MR. A: Let me tell you this, nobody has ever found an answer to it.

MR. E: Sure, why not?

MR. H: Are you familiar with this problem?

MR. A: Why I'm me?

MR. H: Why you're you and why you weren't made someone else?

MR. A: I'm me by heredity and by environmental factors. I was born in a certain house for a certain number of years with two people, one people, et cetera (sic), under a certain environment; that's why I'm me.

MR. D: So you do know the answer.

MR. A: I thought he was asking something else.

MR. H: It seems all these major philosophers and theologians—do they call it a double psychosis, Doctor?

DOCTOR: Somehow I don't understand those words.

MR. H: In reading this Martin Buber's *I and Thou* relation, he mentioned this.

DOCTOR: I don't know the works of Buber, sorry.

MR. D: I started *I and Thou*. I got a quarter of the way through and that was the end of *I and Thou*.

MR. H: It made me uncomfortable to read these thoughts. I would be uncomfortable to be confronted with this type of thought.

MR. A: I never read Buber. I've read most of the other philosophers at some time but what they were concerned with was not I-Thou relations, as you can call it—as he calls it.

MR. H: It doesn't bother me now. It's funny, there were times it bothered me but not now talking about it.

DOCTOR: Mr. I, what's your first name?

MR. I: (Says name.)

MR. A: See, what is a problem perhaps is questions perhaps such as, "What are you?"

MR. H: Yeah.

MR. A: What is the real you? This is a question. But for that again I recommend a Philo course.

MR. L: There are so many "you's," there is not just one constant mood.

MR. A: There are so many different interpretations of this that it doesn't even pay to go into it.

MR. D: I was going to say he did me too proud, but I don't mind; it's all in good fun. I'm thick-skinned anyhow.

MR. L: That's the whole thing; I don't want to be the me that I am now. I want to be—

MR. H: A different me, huh?

MR. L: I don't know. I want to be the same person.

MR. D: I think now is the time to take your poll and see if everyone would join in on the poll.

MR. A: Did Dr. F call you? (Mr. A leaves the identity problem by moving to a discussion of an imminent reality. A surgeon had recommended that he have a herniorrhaphy. Mr. A wanted to make sure his epilepsy was kept under control during his hospitalization. Although he continued to be somewhat immature, Mr. A had managed to enter college and do honors work in philosophy during his treatment in the group. His pneumoencephalogram showed a dilated ventricle on the right. His mother had had a psychotic breakdown requiring her to be hospitalized for six months when Mr. A was seven.)

DOCTOR: No.

MR. A: He said he was going to call you.

DOCTOR: No, he didn't.

MR. A: He wants me to have an operation, and you know; unless I get your okay on it and unless you talk to him, I'm not going through anything.

DOCTOR: Yeah. Well, I'll try to remember to call him.

MR. D: Is this often, this thing that you mentioned?

MR. H: Thoughts like this make me think I'll lose control of myself. And slowly and surely I come to realize that I don't lose control of myself. (The fear of loss of control is tied up with the identity problem. An identity implies an organization that has a pattern which includes control of the organization of the personality.)

MR. I: Come to think of it, I usually have things like that on my mind. I ask myself questions, just as you, "What are you?" and so forth. But I find that may be because I'm bored, the atmosphere that I live in, the civilization, the way people do things. I feel that I'm not really a part of it, I feel I should be different, doing something else, because I don't feel that people the way we're living now in the city, the way people adapt themselves to certain ideas, we're not more or less free, we're more or less hung together. (Mr. I speaks of another aspect of the identity problem, the feeling of isolation. He's not like the others and therefore cannot belong to their group.)

MR. A: Where do you live, incidentally?

MR. I: (a borough, a section of the borough.)

MR. D: Don't you think living in the sort of society that you do you're bound to have certain restraints? Everybody would like to be a bit different from what they are but—

MR. I: I think I feel it more as the years go by. I think I should change my atmosphere, perhaps the people I live around, and so forth. I don't know, this is just a thought that comes to me.

MR. D: In other words, to make yourself freer?

MR. I: Right.

MR. D: Do you think there is such a place, where one can be free absolutely? Free in what sense, by the way?

MR. I: Not in the sense of, say, working five days a week. We know we have to work to eat.

MR. D: That's what he meant by the society we live in.

MR. I: Right. You have to work to eat, but I don't see why a person couldn't do less work and still have the same amount of pay.

MR. D: If everybody had that idea, there would be less accomplished in the long run. We would strive to do less and less and less and we would do nothing in the long run.

MR. I: Well, some people would, of course, want to do less and less and get away with it. But if we would all adjust ourselves—

MR. A: Such a society exists only in the minds of certain idealists.

MR. D: Who is to make the adjustment? I see you doing less and I want to do less than you do. I feel I would become envious of this great ideal that you have. There are very few people that would want to continue working. And yet you do have to eat.

MR. I: I don't mean stop completely, but I don't want to overdo it either.

MR. D: You see, they have cut back the work week; they're continually doing it.

MR. E: Just enough to let you get two jobs.

MR. D: Well, if you want to, sure. (This long discussion of "who and what you are" has exhausted itself. No intervention of the therapist was necessary. Now Mr. L takes up his obsessions.)

MR. L: I can see myself worrying about this dog now. I know I'm going to worry about it. It doesn't make any sense and I don't think I can stop.

MR. D: Why don't you equate the dog with the oil problem that you had? Nothing happened there. Why don't you equate it with the dog?

MR. L: I saw him this Tuesday, I saw him last Tuesday, and if I see—

MR. H: Don't you believe the doctor, what he says?

DOCTOR: But that's not really the problem. (This attempt to begin to look at the form rather than the content failed.)

MR. L: But what is the problem? What causes me to worry about all these things?

MR. J: But didn't you say the dog—

MR. L: If it's not that, it's something else.

MR. J: Didn't you say when you were small you used to like dogs?

MR. L: I used to love them. I used to play with them all the time. I used to get bites but as I get older—

DOCTOR: In other words, when he got older—

MR. D: Not trying to usurp your position as the doctor, it seems he'll always find something to worry about.

MR. L: That's what impresses me, I always find something to worry about. Sometimes I wish I was a moron so I wouldn't think of so many things.

MR. D: What makes you think they don't think?

MR. A: They would think of their ignorance.

MR. E: Don't you wish you were a genius so you could think of more?

MR. L: No, I wouldn't be living if I was a genius.

MR. H: The more you talk about things the more I recall these things in my own case too.

MR. D: How did you overcome all your worry, assuming you did to a certain extent?

MR. H: I don't think I've overcome it to a certain extent; that's why I'm here.

DOCTOR: But I wonder why nobody picked him up when he said he enjoyed the art course when he forced himself to concentrate. (Another attempt to get the group to examine what Mr. L reports was more successful.)

MR. L: Sometimes I feel if I force myself to concentrate I pour other things out of my mind when I have to.

MR. H: So it can be done.

MR. L: I guess it can.

MR. D: Why don't you push yourself a little more?

MR. L: I only seem to push myself when there is a deadline.

MR. D: Look at it this way; you say you worry all the time. Isn't that enough of a deadline?

MR. L: Yes.

MR. D: So why don't you push yourself?

MR. L: I don't know, I don't seem to get anywhere. Even during the transit strike when I was sleeping over, I wasn't studying and I wasn't worrying.

MR. D: Then you weren't pushing yourself, were you?

MR. L: I only pushed myself when there was only two hours left; then I started studying. The dealines seem to come closer and closer; it used to be a week or more.

DOCTOR: Why do you think nobody picked that up when he talked about it? (This question is really aimed at getting the group to try to look more closely at what is said.)

MR. D: I don't think we may be as all knowledgeable that we could associate it at the time it was said. I myself, in spite of the fact that I have a degree, honorary as it is, conferred on me by Mr. A—

MR. A: Oh, oh, is that what you mean?

MR. D: —am not aware what to look for. All right, I think we'll let it die. I'll give up my degree, how is that?

MR. A: We will consider the resignation.

MR. D: Thank you.

MR. H: This is one of the most enjoyable sessions. (The patients have begun to look at what they are doing. This examination of their resistances continues.)

DOCTOR: Do you have something to say, Mr. J?

MR. J: No, it's just that if it's something to do with that, I can't see it because I probably have the same problem.

MR. E: I think I do have the same problem. That's why I mentioned it earlier to him. That's why I projected it onto him.

MR. L: It's amazing. I thought my problem was unique.

DOCTOR: It is. It is.

MR. H: Let's start a unique club here.

MR. L: I'm always so ashamed to talk like this; it just bothers me. I don't know.

MR. D: Mr. J and I discussed this thing in the first session where I sat in, where he had to overcome something and I told him I had the same thing on the job.

MR. L: The only time I would really like to talk would be after I would overcome something, and as I think back on it, I could recall it but it's so hard to talk about what you're thinking about and it sounds so stupid to you; just imagine how stupid it must sound to everybody else. It's so hard for me to come here every week; every week I say I'm not going to come. There are times I do and times I don't. I'm just ashamed, ashamed of coming here altogether. (Mr. L sums up his resistant attitudes toward the group psychotherapy. The other patients take this up in terms of their own feelings.)

MR. H: Does anyone else feel that way?

MR. D: I don't.

MR. H: I sometimes feel that way too.

MR. T: Feel ashamed of coming here?

MR. H: Well, no, the whole idea that I should be afflicted, because this is part of it, part of having some type of affliction.

MR. L: Well, something like what you have I wouldn't be ashamed to talk about.

MR. D: I have many other things.

MR. L: Well, I don't know of any other things. But what you talked about so far I wouldn't be ashamed to talk about.

MR. D: I've come here with the idea that if I am ashamed I'm going to overcome it. I am pushing myself to a certain extent.

MR. L: So am I.

MR. D: It isn't easy to say certain things that I've said here; they're intimate. And yet I say if I'm coming here, I will.

DOCTOR: Are you still taking the medicine?

MR. D: Yes.

DOCTOR: Why don't you cut down on it, omitting every other night, or something like that.

MR. D: I was thinking of that.

DOCTOR: You're not taking it in the day?

MR. D: No. I have cut down on the phenobarb. By the way, this headache; I tried it after the last session after it came on, and I didn't take anything and surprisingly, it didn't last at all.

DOCTOR: But if you had taken something it would have made it better, this *post hoc propter hoc* thing.

MR. T: Speaking of headaches, I haven't had a headache since my wife left.

MR. A: Incidentally, I drew a couple of conclusions from last meeting and two goals I set up for myself. The first thing, I guess you were right when you said that it must have been a Freudian slip of some sort, when I said I had to hate someone and you said he surely does but he doesn't understand it. And I think I drew the conclusion from that later when I was coming home that I have to hate someone as the substitution for the hate of myself. And also another conclusion that I drew from the last meeting— I don't remember how I drew this conclusion—

DOCTOR: You did it by calculus.

MR. A: Yeah, perhaps. Perhaps I took an adding machine.

DOCTOR: Well, what's the other?

MR. A: The other conclusion that I came to was that I have a tendency too much to attempt to impress, let's say, that I am too, too much trying to impress people to, you know, have a favorable image of me, and this tendency to impress tends to be self-destructive because the methods that I employ tend to produce the opposite result.

MR. L: You feel everything you have to say has to be provocative or exceptionally stimulating.

MR. A: That's the point, that's what I was trying to say, but that's not good; that's not what I should do.

MR. L: Yeah, because I listen to people talking sometimes and they're not really talking about anything at all, not trying to impress anyone, not trying to tell someone something they don't already know, just making conversation, not saying anything.

MR. A: I guess I have to of necessity make up for what I feel are my own inadequacies and there is one thing that I remember that's perhaps one of the best pieces of advice that I've ever gotten. Before I left the old clinic about three years ago, the man who had been working with me there told me something I guess which I'm lately coming around to understand more and more: Don't try to destroy your own attempts at socializing. That's a paraphrase.

DOCTOR: Uh-huh.

MR. A: But that was the general idea of it. And I think lately, you know, I've been trying to be a little more conscious of my actions.

DOCTOR: I'm not sure that I would agree with your arithmetic, but I would generally agree with your conclusions.

MR. A: You would generally agree with my conclusions but you wouldn't agree with my arithmetic?

DOCTOR: No. (The transference reactions in the previous discussions are obviously related to the positive feelings these patients have toward the therapist. To show great pleasure on hearing them would be likely to provoke sychophantic, therapeutically useless discussion.)

MR. A: Yeah, yeah, I understand.

DOCTOR: How is that for being mysterious?

MR. A: No, it's very simple.

DOCTOR: No, I don't follow his logic in coming to these conclusions but I subscribe to the sum of them.

MR. A: He doesn't agree with what I call the causes but he does agree with what I call the effects.

DOCTOR: QED. This is getting pretty sad. It's come to that. But there is some phrase for this, but I don't remember.

MR. L: I'm lost. QED?

DOCTOR: That means—that's an abbreviation for something or other that means what's to be proved has been proved.

MR. A: Oh, *qua ergo*, or something?

MR. L: Oh, I see.

DOCTOR: A guy comes to the blackboard with figures, you know, that's QED. But never mind, this is getting pretty dense. Let's stop, that's enough for tonight.

*   *   *

Notes on Session 1

Problems about being a husband and father, which relate to the identity of each patient, are discussed. The identity committee aspect of the group occurs in the discussion of Mr. T's separation from his wife. The masculine role of the protector and provider is spontaneously delineated in the group discussion.

The problems of epilepsy are coincidental in Mr. E and Mr. T.

The problems of growing up and identity definition related to dependence-independence of parents are explored.

The intervention by the therapist to prevent Mr. T from giving Mr. L some girls' phone numbers was for the purpose of keeping the work of the group aimed at accomplishing some worthwhile change in Mr. L's mode of operation, rather than to give him the answers. The therapy should help him to learn how to solve the problems himself.

Patients see they have things in common and can work together. (Mr. H says to Mr. J, "I have the same problem.")

Mr. A speaks of what he got from preceding sessions. He examines himself and Mr. L compares himself.

The joking references to arithmetic and conclusions at the end of the session were designed to keep the discussion open and relieve the tension in the group. This includes relieving the tension provoked in the therapist during the handling of the negative, then positive transferences and resistances.

Session 2

At this session Mr. A, Mr. J, and Mr. I did not appear. Mr. F, a borderline phobic who had missed the previous session, had returned.

Mr. D: I didn't take the alternate days that you suggested. I wasn't able to start it this week. (Mr. D took phenobarbital and tranquilizers. He glaringly alternated compliance and failure to follow directions. However, he improved steadily.)

Doctor: You decided to continue taking the medicine every day?

Mr. D: Well, for this week at least. Would there be any advantage to cutting down the dose or don't you think so?

Doctor: Oh, it might be done.

Mr. D: Do you think I ought to do that or—

Doctor: You take a capsule, don't you?

Mr. D: Right. How do I take a lesser capsule?

Doctor: There is one smaller than that. It's a pretty small dose but it can be done.

Mr. D: Well, there is a 75 and there is a 30. I'm taking the 150.

Doctor: Oh, I keep thinking you're taking the 75.

Mr. D: No. We started off with the 75 and then went to 150. You think I should take the 75?

Doctor: All right, we'll give you the 75 then.

Mr. D: Right, and then if I'm feeling all right, I'll try alternating.

Mr. E: What are you laughing at?

Doctor: What am I what?

Mr. E: Laughing at.

Doctor: I was writing the prescription and I saw this thing going over there and it's your foot. (This amusement was partly a reaction to the annoyance at not being able to keep up with Mr. D and what he did with the medications prescribed.)

Mr. E: Oh, well.

Doctor: How are you, Mr. L?

Mr. L: I'm okay now. I've been all right the last few days. I don't know, there is one thing, something I didn't worry about, there was nothing—I just—I couldn't make myself worry and then I felt guilty that I didn't. It was a crazy feeling.

Doctor: What do you mean?

Mr. L: Because there was nothing at all to worry about, but if I followed the pattern I would have been worried. I don't know. I was in my art class last Friday and we're doing skeletons; we're drawing skeletons in the hope to improve, you know, drawing the figure, you know, skulls. First it was the human skull and as we were drawing I was thinking, I was talking to a few of my friends and the friends I had in the class before—see, it's the same teacher I had the first term of art and this is the second term of art and they all got "A's" and I only got a "B plus." So I was just thinking maybe I should go up to this teacher and ask her why she didn't give me an "A," but I felt it was kind of a stupid thing to do, so like after the class ended, you know, I was hanging around a little while; I was going to ask her, and then as I was hanging around—see, we had different things, we had skeletons, skulls of human beings, a skull of a ground hog, skull of birds, the skull of a dog, so I was fooling around with the skull of the dog and I cut myself on one of the teeth because I was a little nervous and fidgety when I was going to ask her that, you know, and I didn't think of anything at the time and then I asked her and she said, well, you know, maybe you can get an "A" this term. Just as long as I asked her I felt better. And then later on in the afternoon I started thinking about—I don't know what I was thinking. I was getting a little bit nervous, but then I stopped myself. That was it. I thought about it a little once in awhile during the week but I stopped, you know, I just figured it's just so stupid, I got to think straight. I mean, I'm not that stupid; I just have to snap out of it. (Mr. L expresses the idea that he is not himself without worries. This self-image is taken up in the group.)

DOCTOR: What do you think of this, Mr. E?

MR. E: Well, you know, I find it extremely interesting.

DOCTOR: Well, that's my favorite noncommittal remark, you know.

MR. E: No, extremely.

DOCTOR: Oh, excuse me, that's right, it isn't noncommittal when you say extremely.

MR. E: Exactly what I should say now, why do I find it interesting—

DOCTOR: Extremely interesting.

MR. E: Why, it just is a sort of a fragment which kind of might be part of a pattern which at times I feel I might be fitting into. (Mr. E correctly speaks of Mr. L's reaction as a pattern of thought and symptomatic.)

DOCTOR: You mean you're catching it from Mr. J?

MR. E: No, it's—not necessarily. I might be completely misinterpreting it.

MR. L: He's felt he's had somewhat similar experiences maybe. I mean, you know, basically.

MR. E: Well, just reluctance, for example, to ask your art teacher.

MR. L: Oh.

MR. E: This is just the one main thing. And I'm gradually, well, I've been looking for jobs. I'm gradually getting over a certain reluctance I have just to approach and ask people aynthing; that is, if I'm applying for a job, I'm, one, sort of reluctant to walk in and ask. It's very difficult for me to sell my personality. I'm reluctant to ask people for recommendations, and so forth, reluctant to infringe upon people if they might be busy and overdoing this. There are other things, but I'll leave it go at that.

DOCTOR: Does this have anything to do with anybody else?

MR. F: Him being reluctant to ask things? I think some of us go through that. I also—even though maybe we're qualified for certain things, we hesitate to, we feel maybe we'll be turned down or someone might say something, so we just don't do it at all. Maybe that has to do with the whole personality pattern of our whole life and these are just fragments of it, just afraid of situations to begin with. (The phobic basis of symptoms is alluded to. This is taken up in the subsequent discussion.)

MR. L: See, I'm thinking maybe one incident has some sort of a bearing on another. Like if I wasn't worried or thinking about asking this professor something, maybe I wouldn't have worried about—wouldn't have been nervous about the other thing, or maybe I would have, I don't know. I'm just wondering if one thing has a bearing on another.

MR. D: I think that to a point everybody suffers from a bit of apprehension at one time or another but the thing that I have found, at least as far as I'm concerned, is to realize that some of the fears are quite groundless and that a great deal of the worrying is done before the actual situation happens. I think this is about the third time I must have said that. I think I say this about every evening that we meet, and each successive time that you're faced with the situation, it becomes a little easier to face up to it.

MR. L: Well, like approaching people, there are times when

I say I'll force myself and for a long time I won't be afraid of approaching someone but if I stop for awhile, for quite awhile, then it's hard for me to get back into it again. But I don't think that's my main problem. It's these—I don't know, it's a fear of diseases, the major problem that's been recurring and hasn't gone away.

Mr. D: But let's take any one of the problems, it's still the same things; you were worried about speaking to the teacher.

Mr. L: Yeah, just to tell her.

Mr. D: Were you worried about the outcome, about what she would say, or the idea of going up there?

Mr. L: I thought it was stupid to go up and ask someone something about the term before.

Mr. D: Why?

Mr. L: I just thought it was stupid; and it was stupid. Like with this problem of being afraid of animals, when I was young I used to play with—they used to be my best friends. I'd have this dog named——you know, these various dogs I'd play with in the park and I'd get a few friends together and we'd have a great time. I was to the doctor about six times when I was little, you know, with these dog bites. Once I almost had stitches but they didn't require it. I still have a little scar on my leg.

Doctor: How are you, Mr. K? (This intervention was made to interrupt Mr. L, who was using his tale for the secondary gain of the attention and sympathy of the group, rather than examining his thinking, and also to give Mr. K a chance to talk. It did not stop Mr. L, who continued after the interruption. The resistance aspect of Mr. L's verbiage was taken up in the next intervention by the therapist. The resistance interpretation was more fruitful.)

Mr. K: Fine.

Mr. L: But as I was saying, when I was young it didn't bother me. When I grew up it started worrying me that dogs that weren't even biting me were biting me, and I was going to get sick and it was just like a delayed reaction and it still stuck with me, and even a skeleton of a dog, it reminded me of it and it reminded me of a time a dog bit me and that even got me nervous, just scratching myself on the teeth of a skeleton, just the thought of it got me nervous, petrified because the doctor tried to instill a fear in me not to go near an animal and I just wouldn't listen to him and then later on it just—

DOCTOR: Well, you have to watch out for these doctors; they'll mess you up if you aren't careful.

MR. L: It's in me; I didn't listen to him before and I had more sense when I was young.

DOCTOR: Well, we doctors are pretty dangerous, you know.

MR. L: It wasn't his fault; it was my fault. I don't even think it was anything he said.

DOCTOR: It may have been something he said.

MR. L: Was it? Why would I think of it later in life instead of then? It didn't affect me then.

MR. F: He told you something to do?

MR. L: Just keep away from them, don't get near them, even a pinprick you might get rabies, or something. He was telling me first to keep me away from them because he didn't want to keep doctoring up my scars. And another thing I have, I feel if I don't—like even to apply for a job or to approach someone, or anything, if I don't do it right away, I have to do something— it's just if I don't do it I'll get so mad at myself it will just be awful. If I feel I should do something and I don't do it, just forget it! I just can't rest until I do it. And I just don't do it right away. I make myself suffer first and then I do it.

MR. E: What do you mean?

MR. L: Anything, just to ask someone for a job, or something. It may seem stupid, like I ask someone for a job eight hours a week, it will just seem stupid, because they employ people full-time as a rule. And then I'll wait around for a couple of days and I won't do it and I wait a couple of days and I do it, instead of doing it right away.

DOCTOR: Why do you wait awhile? (This represented an effort to get Mr. L to look at himself. The next intervention by the therapist was to try to get opinions from the other patients about Mr. L.)

MR. L: I don't know, I just don't do it.

DOCTOR: Do you know why he waits, Mr. D?

MR. D: I think he wants to punish himself. My reaction is

quite the opposite of Mr. L's. When I have something distasteful to do, I get it over with very quickly.

MR. L: See, if I get it over with very quickly then there is no problem.

MR. D: Well, then, that's it then. As I said, I really can't say what it is you do it but the thing to do if you know there is no problem is to get rid of it.

MR. L: I always think of myself as doing something foolish.

MR. D: Yes, you said that several times.

MR. L: And that holds me back. Asking a perfectly simple question seems so foolish.

DOCTOR: You're afraid you might not make a good impression? (The phobic aspect of the behavior is clearly stated.)

MR. L: Maybe, but if the person doesn't know me—I don't know what it is, that might be it.

MR. D: Why should you think everything you do is stupid?

MR. L: I don't know.

(The following group discussion involves Mr. L's symptoms and at times shows the symptomatic behavior of the other patients.)

MR. D: There is nothing so wrong in asking about a mark. It's something you don't think might have been quite fair. It's done all the time, by the way. My daughter does it, and as a matter of fact, she's been encouraged to do it if she feels the mark might have been a mistake; the teacher may have made a mistake. Not to go up every five minutes.

MR. L: Well, as I said before, I still think it's stupid.

MR. D: Why?

MR. L: A "B plus" or an "A," what's the big deal?

MR. D: Well, you can rationalize anything.

MR. L: Well, it's not such a big deal.

MR. D: It's big enough if it annoys you.

MR. E: Well, except that you have a better chance, you realize, with this, than you would the difference between a "D" and an "F" because the fellow wouldn't do that without a good reason to start with.

MR. L: The thing is you can't change the marks after they're in anyway. I mean, this is the next term already, the second week in the term. It just seemed like a stupid question; I didn't want to bother her with a stupid question.

Mr. K: Stupid in whose eyes, your eyes?

Mr. L: Mine, yeah.

Mr. K: Then what's the big deal if it's a stupid question?

Mr. L: Because it bothered me if I didn't ask.

Mr. E: In an art class, how do you feel about being very mark conscious anyway?, since it is perhaps a more nebulous field, where achievement isn't—

Mr. L: Yeah, it's achievement that's the mark. I'm not worried about it. I don't really care. I just felt bad when I asked her. Just the idea of asking her; I didn't care what her answer was. It's just forcing myself to do something I felt I should do, even though I thought it was stupid. It makes a lot of sense.

Mr. E: You know, it's very interesting, back to sort of passiveness. First of all, I was, one, interested when you said you found certain things distasteful, because I think emotionally, or however you would term the word, I don't really find anything distasteful. I'd just take a more clinical attitude towards this, whatever it might be. If I'm walking on a highway and a car passes me within a couple of inches at sixty miles an hour, I just continue walking down the highway. In a sense I won't necessarily look around; it's just something that happens and it's already happened.

Mr. D: Supposing it's coming towards you and swerves away?

Mr. E: I might feel some emotion.

Mr. D: Just some?

Mr. E: Yes.

Mr. D: You mean it wouldn't rankle you at all?

Mr. E: Not necessarily. It might, but it hasn't in the past. I suppose if I thought there was intent it might.

Mr. D: If he was coming toward you and suddenly swerved away that might preclude a certain amount of intent.

Mr. E: But it's interesting in job interviews, people know right away, generally speaking in about two or three minutes— suppose I'm looking for a job in a company, they'll know, one, I don't have the personality for sales just like that, which is quite honest, fine, good. I don't get into a job I'm not capable for.

But it's a little bit beguiling to know it's really all that obvious, the personality.

MR. L: When you talk about job interviews, I seem to like them when I actually get in the office and start talking, because I remember during the summer I did that a lot. I wanted just to work during the summer and I would say that I would work, you know, make a life career out of it. And I had to make up references and things I did and I sort of enjoyed acting, pretending I was, I don't know, sort of like a different type of person. I seem to like that.

MR. E: Pretending you're a different person than you are?

MR. L: Yeah, pretending. I don't know, I was different. Like once I felt very cocky one day, I went in for an interview. I had to take a test. I did well on the test. It was three weeks before I had to go back to school because I lost another job and I didn't want to just hang around the street. I did but I just couldn't. I hung around for two days and I felt so disgusted with myself I just couldn't. But then I looked for work again. And you know, I was talking to this guy and I was telling him what a great worker I am and it would be an asset to the company to have me and it was just too much and he was saying, gee, you're very strong-willed and set in your ways. I really got a kick out of that interview.

MR. E: Well, did you get the job?

MR. L: No. Well, he checked my references. He said, "You have the job but let me check your references first." I didn't have any really. Then I went to the temporary agency. I got a job there for two weeks. I was working for them before and then I tried it again. (The underlying phobic basis of the behavior has become apparent.)

* * *

(Here the verbatim notes of the last session were read back.*)

MR. E: What do you mean by emotional liability? I mean, you said it.

---

* According to the technique described in "The Use of Verbatim Minutes in Group Psychotherapy: The Development of a 'Readback' Technique." (*op. cit.*)

DOCTOR: Lability or labile, flexible or changeable. Shall we wake up Mr. L? (Mr. L had avoided listening to the reading of the notes of the previous session by falling asleep. After the readback the therapist allows himself and the group to be distracted from the notes of the previous session when Mr. L shifts the topic to his sleep.)

MR. L: It's comfortable.

DOCTOR: Pardon?

MR. L: It was very comfortable.

DOCTOR: Oh, I'm sorry to disturb you.

MR. L: I mentioned something about when I was sleeping over during the transit strike; I think I was worried about something then too. I was debating whether or not to apply for a job in the library, or something, and it was sort of at the end of the term and I wanted to apply for the beginning of the next term and I didn't know my program. I don't know, I was thinking about that and it was getting me nervous, until I finally didn't do anything. This thought came to me. I'm always worrying about something. I notice when—about a year ago I used to sleep more like on a train. Even last term—no, term before last, at least then I could stop worrying because I fell asleep. Lately, I don't know, very rarely do I do it. I don't think I should because it's just wasting my time. (He is aware of the avoidance of "worry" by falling asleep.)

MR. E: Do what?

MR. L: Falling asleep.

MR. E: Do you want to fall asleep?

MR. L: What?

MR. E: Do you find, for example, supposing you have to do some school work—

MR. L: Yeah.

MR. E: —and you feel so upset that you figure during a twenty-four period you're going to have to sleep anyway, you figure maybe if you sleep now you can do it later?

MR. L: Yeah, sometimes.

MR. E: Does it change your eating habits? (Mr. E connects sleeping and eating.)

MR. L: Well, I don't stay up all night.

MR. E: Do you have any eating problems? Do you eat more?

MR. L: If I'm very nervous. I know when I don't eat regularly it bothers me. If I don't do things regularly it bothers me. Anything really. If I don't eat regularly or do what I'm supposed to be doing, at least if I go through motions I feel much better.

DOCTOR: He's the man they aim the (a laxative) advertising at, you see. (This comment was exploratory. Mr. L did not respond with any talk about his feelings about bowel movements. Mr. E took it up in terms of his social anxiety.)

MR. E: Yeah. You reckon they also aim the other advertisements, like halitosis, and deodorants, and so forth and so on, and you get—when you get anxiety about personal relationships, why don't those girls seem to be approachable? Or for the girls, I suppose it's the reverse, why don't they approach me? It really in a sense must be a fairly generalized thing in the population at large, that these advertisers are exploiting, is that not—

DOCTOR: What do you think, Mr. H?

MR. H: Sure. Because I understand they go through quite an extensive study before they spend all this money on advertising. Very definitely there must be people with these problems. Is this the point that you wanted to make?

MR. E: Yeah, right, right.

MR. H: Sure.

MR. E: I'm glad you make that point. They begin to stiffen my resistance to things after awhile. I mean it was very difficult for me to stop cigarettes but finally when I came back and I started watching television for the first time in a couple of years, it was so sickening, you know, the obvious play, that I stopped— also last week it was willpower, and this kind of thing. I tried previously—but I feel like a sucker if I actually do what they tell me to do. I've almost reversed it. I tend to avoid the specific products that I've heard.

MR. H: There must be an awful lot of suckers around because this seems to work.

MR. F: Do you do that? That's interesting. In other words, if you see something on TV and they're advertising, you won't buy it then?

Mr. H: In defiance, right?

Mr. F: Because I do the reverse sometimes.

Mr. E: But I'm not terribly conscious of this all the time. But generally it brings out an adverse reaction. (Mr. E's fear of conformity is apparent.)

Mr. F: But you want to defy them; you don't want to do it.

Mr. E: No, it's a question of taste, I suppose.

Mr. F: That's very interesting. If I have a favorite program I'm watching on TV, I say that's the brand I smoke, and this program happens to be one of the top shows and I get a certain pleasure out of that, which is just the reverse of what you seem to be doing.

Mr. E: I figure if they have to push it that hard, it's not any good.

Mr. F: Maybe they're not pushing it. They're not that loud. It depends on what they're selling.

Mr. E: Generally they're more creative than the program, I'll agree with you there. They're nice to watch as a work of art, not to have it motivate your behavior.

Mr. H: I don't know if this has anything to do with this, but do you recall this (a TV commercial)? It's a fabulous commercial. I read somewhere it wasn't selling beer. They had to use a jingle approach, so they're cautious of this and they know when they're selling the people and they're not.

Doctor: You wait for the claque.

Mr. D: There are some instances where you wait for the claque and then go ahead and do it.

Mr. F: But what makes them do it first?

Mr. D: They're less inhibited than you.

Mr. F: Well, this is the thing.

Mr. E: It's an anonymous job really.

Mr. D: You're talking about being members of a claque, is that right?

Mr. E: Yes. You don't have to be inhibited at all; it's a crowd.

Doctor: They do have to. They have to be quiet at the time and not let other people applaud at the wrong time.

MR. E: This is what I meant by bad manners. There may be some point where you're not supposed to clap and if you're unsure you won't do it so you won't make a mistake. (The phobic aspect is referred to by his saying "if you're unsure.")

DOCTOR: *You* won't but the others might. (The annoyance of the therapist at Mr. L is displaced to Mr. E.)

MR. D: I don't know if you're familiar with it, there is a great pause in Mendelssohn's Violin Concerto, a terrific pause between the movements, and invariably there is a smattering of applause at this spot and all those in the know look around and say ha, ha, you goofed.

MR. L: It's interesting what you said about buying things on TV. It just seems you're following the crowd, following along with everybody else.

DOCTOR: What's wrong with that? (To raise questions about their fears of losing themselves by conforming and acquiring an identity.)

MR. L: I don't know. It seems like in the morning on the stations, everyone is on their toes, waiting for the train to come along, so they can devour—get a seat. I don't like to be part of the mob.

DOCTOR: Why not?

MR. L: Because at the moment it seems to me they're animals like.

MR. D: Supposing you're driven with the obsession of getting a seat?

MR. L: Well, I feel the same way.

MR. D: Do you want to sit down badly?

MR. L: Yeah.

MR. D: But not badly enough so you will join the mob in the rush for the seat.

MR. L: I don't do that much now because I don't go in the rush hour. But last year I had to go every morning in the rush hour. In the beginning I did it, but after awhile I had a reluctance in doing it. I don't like to join part of the mob because I don't like to become part of the mob.

MR. E: Do you ever take the same attitude toward yourself?

MR. L: What do you mean?

MR. E: You look at what you're doing; did I do that?, is it me? (Reflects the identity problem.)

MR. L: Sometimes.

MR. H: Yeah.

MR. E: You do?

MR. H: Yeah.

MR. E: I don't. I just asked the question.

MR. H: Yeah, like kind of an introspection.

MR. L: Yeah, I may say that when he'd be reading the notes, or something, it doesn't sound like what I said. (The identity problems and the recognition of reality provoked by the readback is emphasized here. Mr. L was "playing possum" and not asleep.)

DOCTOR: You did.

MR. D: Don't you remember saying it when you hear it?

MR. L: Yeah, but certain things don't sound like what I say.

MR. D: I noticed something as everyone was talking. I notice for the most part everyone here is greatly given to introspection; I mean a great deal of introspection. We're pretty much involved with ourselves. And I wonder why this is. I think when you asked why we didn't pick up Mr. L in what he said, I think that was indicative of the fact that we all had his problem, to a degree.

MR. E: Hold it now. I mean the whole thing is designed in doing this sort of thing, it is not? I mean, I'll accept your premise to a certain extent. (The effect of the readback is noted.)

MR. D: What I said is we are involved in introspection to a great degree, which might be considered the norm, which is a very wide way of putting it. In other words, I don't think that people who function in a way that is considered normal—again I have to use this word normal because normal is many different things to many people—think of themselves a great deal less, aren't concerned with every pain, aren't concerned with every incident, don't magnify the slightest things and make a big thing out of them. They are less introspective than we are here. We are very involved in what is worrying us.

MR. H: Is this so, doctor?

DOCTOR: Well, is it for you?

MR. H: It might be. He seems to be hitting on something good.

MR. L: I tried to stop that by thinking of other people and I think I started with my parents and I started worrying about them.

MR. D: Do you find that you think of yourself to a large extent?

MR. L: When I start thinking of someone else, I'll get just as nervous about them as I will about me.

MR. D: I was speaking to the gentleman next to you. Do you find that you think of yourself to a large extent?

MR. K: I think of myself. I have absolutely no idea of what the norm is.

MR. D: That's what I mean. By the norm I mean a great deal more than—

MR. K: Again, I have no way of telling. I think of myself, sure. Sometimes I don't. If I'm reading my paper I'm not thinking of myself.

MR. E: Tonight, for example, would you be thinking of yourself so much that you have withdrawn from the conversation?

MR. K: I don't know. No, I don't think I'm thinking so much of myself. The reason I don't say much in these things, I don't think I have anything to say that's pertinent to anything.

MR. E: So you don't think your problems are sort of worthy of consideration but on the other hand, you do because that's why you're here.

MR. K: I don't see talking about advertising, very truthfully, how it's going to help me. I can't get excited about it.

MR. L: Yeah, but just try it first and work into it and see what happens.

MR. D: That's what I meant. That's what I meant when I spoke about introspection. I meant about devoting a great deal of thought to what you think is bothering you.

MR. H: Sure.

MR. K: I very truthfully have no idea of what my problems are. I have a couple of ideas about the symptoms. (This perceptive statement should lead the group to a better understanding of the relation of symptoms to problems. It doesn't.)

MR. D: Well, do you think about them?

MR. K: No. I'm almost completely convinced I'm the only sane person in the whole world. I've come here; it wasn't my idea; it was my parents. Again, I'm not going to be the next saint, but obviously there is something wrong with me.

MR. D: Well, from what you said I myself would gather you don't give that much thought to yourself. As far as you're concerned, you don't have too great a problem, I guess.

MR. K: Well, I'm sure there is a problem but I can't put my finger on it.

MR. E: You mean you'd be disappointed if you found out you were as nuts as everybody else?

MR. K: No, I wouldn't be disappointed. I don't know if I should be here, that's all.

MR. D: Did you understand what I was saying?

MR. H: Yes.

DOCTOR: What do you think, Mr. F, do you agree with Mr. D?

MR. F: What you said about everybody else being crazy, sometimes when I get into an argument with my father, I say everybody else is crazy; I'm going to go along with everybody else. Sometimes he wants me to do something but I object to it. I say the whole world is crazy, so why not go along? I don't know if that's what you had in mind.

MR. D: No.

MR. F: Or the bomb is going to fall tomorrow, so why worry about it?

MR. K: Do you mean when you're here you think about your own problems?

MR. D: No. In other words, when you're alone. I don't mean in the context of the meeting that we have here. I mean in general away from here.

MR. X: Don't you think in general anybody that's coming to a meeting like this, there is something that's not exactly right in their life?

MR. D: Yes. I've said that and I feel it too.

MR. X: If you have a headache, you think about your headache. If you have an ingrown toenail, you think about your ingrown toenail. And if the reason you're here is such a disruptive factor in your life, I think the most normal thing in the world is to think about it.

Mr. D: You just said if you have a headache you think about it. Some people have a headache and don't think about it; they don't ascribe anything else to it. They don't wonder how they can get rid of it. They don't wonder whether, like the doctor said, if they take an aspirin, whether the next aspirin will make it go away. They just have a headache and that's all.

Mr. K: But we equate it with whatever emotional problem you have. In other words, a headache—

Doctor: In other words, the only reason you're here is because you love your parents and they want you to come here. (This deliberately distorted review of Mr. K's previous remarks was designed to provoke a clear statement from him of his reasons for coming to the group psychotherapy. In fact, the urging of his father was the strongest motive in his attending. However, Mr. K did recognize the real reasons for his getting the treatment.)

Mr. K: No, I'm convinced there is something wrong somewhere. In other words, things aren't smooth. I don't know what's wrong. I have no idea.

Mr. D: Have I made myself clear?

Mr. E: You said we do too much thinking about ourselves.

Mr. F: In the wrong way.

Mr. D: I wouldn't say it's the wrong way. We devote too much time to ourselves in introspection.

Mr. F: That's not too bad. Let's say if a man wanted to earn money and that's what he thought about.

Mr. D: But supposing we devote the same amount of thought to trivia, if it really isn't that important.

Mr. K: Isn't that your answer? You don't give that much importance to trivia.

Mr. D: Let's not say that's the answer. Let's say in my case that's the objective.

Mr. K: I don't follow you. I don't see why you put so much emphasis on what's not important.

Mr. D: I want to get into the end where I place or equate,

not attach the same amount of worry to everything. Let's say I want to have a few gradations in my worrying patterns.

Mr. K: Don't you?

Mr. D: No.

Mr. K: That doesn't seem at all possible. I mean the slightest irritation you worry as much as your own emotional problems?

Mr. D: I take some things that are really trivial, if I stop and think about them, and I worry about them. I worry about a great many things that never happen. I anticipate them happening and when the time comes all the worrying is for naught.

Mr. E: You mean things like worrying about going around the corner, you'll be hit by a car?

Mr. D: No. Things like—well, to cite an example offhand is difficult.

Mr. H: Death?

Mr. D: No. Let's say we spend eight hours a day working; let's say a problem on the job; I anticipate all the pitfalls, all of the stumbling blocks, and yet they suddenly just fade out; they never appear.

Mr. K: But there is a possibility that the worst will happen, right?

Mr. D: Yes, but there are people who don't envision the worst happening. That's exactly what I'm telling you. They don't spend their time worrying about what's going to happen. They just go along and wait for the thing to happen. Suppose you take the opposite effect, where you don't anticipate something going to happen, where you say I'm going to wait until something is going to happen, and then worry.

Mr. K: In other words, you have apprehensions about certain things happening?

Mr. D: I have certain apprehensions about things going to happen. There are people who don't have these apprehensions.

Mr. E: There are, but that's not necessarily an advantage.

Mr. D: Well, I think in my case, not to achieve a complete pattern where I don't worry or anticipate, but to be able to take each problem as it comes up without the anticipatory juggling.

Mr. K: But sometimes you can take steps to avoid something

by anticipating it. (This is the rationalization for phobic behavior.)

MR. D: Lots of times you don't even need to initiate these steps because they never come about.

DOCTOR: Time, time; we have to stop.

* * *

Further Observations on Session 2

Mr. D, a severe obsessive-compulsive, started off in his oppositional way. He had not been able to follow the recommendations about his medication.

Mr. L discussed his own thinking processes and behavior. He had begun some kind of self-evaluation. The therapist promoted some interaction with Mr. E.

Mr. F then compared his *modus operandi* to that of the others. The identity committee effect was in operation.

Mr. D was drawn into the interaction.

The reactions to the notes of the last session reinforced the stimulus of the patients to think about themselves and the group interaction. Their appreciation of the immediate reality was strengthened. The group interaction continued.

Mr. E's contrariness came out and he discussed it as a part of personality.

The phobic quality of Mr. E's behavior become evident.

Mr. L's problems in identity are expressed by his fear of becoming only a part of the mob.

Mr. H participated very little but was alert and responsive to the discussion. He had been concerned with introspection and being passively accepting or actively opposed to advertising.

Mr. E pointed out to Mr. K that his problems and ultimately himself had been "worthy of discussion." Mr. K tried to deny this.

Session 3

This session was attended by five of the six patients who had attended Session 2, Messrs. D, K, E, H and L. Mr. J had returned after missing Session 2.

* * *

MR. E: Free samples? (Referring to drug samples on the

desk. Mr. E was the relative of an important person in contact with the therapist. His somewhat presumptious familiarity added to the difficulties encountered in his treatment.)

DOCTOR: Yeah. Which one do you want   (Hiding one in each hand.) Yeah, I don't know exactly what to do with them. They're hard to get rid of. I used to send them to a doctor who runs a hospital in Africa or I used to give them to somebody who sent it to him, but it got terribly complicated because it had some kind of a special duty to be paid on drugs, all kinds of special declarations to be made, and it got not to be worth the effort. The Africans can go ahead and die while you're filling out the forms and paying the taxes. So I still have them. Hospital pharmacies don't take them any more.

MR. E: I know somebody running a hospital in Indonesia.

DOCTOR: Can you get them in there? It's not easy.

MR. D: I found something very interesting in the medication, while we're talking about them. The 150's seem to cost almost the same as the 75's but then there is a marked decrease when you go down to the 30's. I wonder why.

DOCTOR: Actually the preparations have little to do with the cost. Penicillin costs less than the bottle it comes in now. I don't know about Thorazine.

MR. D: He said something about the preparations. When you get above 75, when you go to 150, it's about the same. The big drop comes below that.

DOCTOR: Well, there are things about the distribution and manufacturing in terms of cost that I don't understand at all.

(Short silence)

MR. L: The silence is deadly. (The silence provoked tension in Mr. L and so he spoke before the other patients. In the preceding session he talked more than any other patient. For him talk seems to be a way of avoiding tension.)

MR. H: I would like to know something. First of all, there are times when I get extremely nervous, tense, about whatever it is that's bothering me. The pills don't seem to work. Well now, there are times when I overcome it and there are times when I can't. I'm just curious if anybody else experiences it and what they do to get rid of it, or do you just wait it out, so to speak?

MR. D: I myself find if I get quite active and take my mind off it, it just disappears, so to speak. Of course, you can't be active all the time.

MR. H: Yeah. If you're sitting at the table and it happens—

MR. D: Yeah, it's true. I think I mentioned that once before. I was just sitting there and this thing came on. It's difficult.

MR. E: How is this manifested?

(Anxiety symptoms are discussed in their various forms in the following exchanges.)

MR. H: I mentioned at one time one of my problems, sometimes I think of all this introspection, sometimes I feel I'll lose control of myself. I know I won't, but somehow I'm afraid I will.

MR. E: Is it physical tension you're speaking of, sort of, that you can't sit still any longer?

MR. H: No, it's not that. It's like an inward type of tension.

MR. E: And you can't relax?

MR. D: But there aren't any overt symptoms?

MR. H: No, no.

MR. D: When I have that happen, I begin to swallow a great deal.

MR. E: Does your mind wander?

MR. H: Yeah.

MR. E: Sort of a fantasy go along with it?

MR. H: You think you're in a sort of a dream and you can't shake it.

MR. E: I've noticed—although not always, but more often than not—that this accompanies what I would consider my periods of tension. Although I must say physically, see, I can lift weights until I'm completely exhausted and it makes no difference.

MR. H: It doesn't help you?

MR. E: To the manifestation of the symptoms, no. It's rather interesting, I have had a very boring routine-type job the last few days, it hasn't bothered me whatsoever at work; absolutely not. Probably the longest period since I've been in this country, in New York, where it hasn't bothered me, where when I have to go home, I have to compose a letter, something that involves maybe decision making, but a really routine stupid job and it doesn't bother me whatsoever. Even during the times I would take a break, have lunch, it doesn't bother me.

MR. H: I find there are times when I can overcome it but yet just the idea that I know that—the anticipating brings it on. You're nodding your head.

MR. D: Yeah. Well, that was what I used to do. I used to take the pills in anticipation of the thing, and I've stopped that, of course.

MR. H: Do you find with the anticipating that could bring it back on?

MR. D: No. I mean when I would take the pill it would have already started. In other words, I wouldn't think of it coming on, it would just come. And then in order to try and check it I would take a pill at that time. Or sometimes if I were going out and I felt it was going to be an exhilerating evening, let's say, I would prepare for it by taking a phenobarb, just to slow myself down. This, of course, I don't think had any great effect.

MR. H: It doesn't help that much?

MR. D: No.

MR. E: This must be something big because on an occasion like that it probably wouldn't bother me at all.

MR. D: Yeah.

MR. H: So you don't find the anticipation of it can bring it on?

MR. D: No. For instance, after the last session where we wound up in quite a heated discussion that we had to terminate, I left here and I was again quite wound up, and I have found that just this type of an animated discussion will have me gulping air and swallowing.

MR. E: Because we agreed, in a sense. It was just a matter over verbal definitions.

MR. D: It wasn't the matter of the content, of the agreement. It was the matter of the stimulation of the discussion. Whether or not I was agreed with didn't enter into it.

MR. E: You were completely involved in it, therefore.

MR. D: I would like to know if there will come a time when I can engage in this type of thing without this happening.

DOCTOR: You mean heated discussion without getting excited?

(The discussions of the group psychotherapy are thought of as anxiety provoking. To relate them to symptoms and problems would be the next step in the treatment.)

MR. D: No. Getting excited and heated discussions without gulping air, without the aftermath, let's say. I want the fun without the aftermath. There was a time, of course, I could do this. This is something that hasn't been going on all my life. It's something that just recently happened.

MR. E: What do you mean by gulping air?

MR. D: I swallow.

MR. E: You don't feel anything with your heart?

MR. D: No.

MR. E: Or in your chest?

MR. D: No.

MR. H: Do you concentrate on your breathing?

MR. D: No, I just gulp air. There is a feeling there is a lump in my throat and I'd like to get rid of it, and the thing I do to get rid of it is just swallow.

MR. H: I've had that rarely.

MR. D: I find that that will happen during the night too after I've gone to sleep. I wake up, start right in.

MR. H: I've had this where I mentioned I would concentrate on my breathing and you think you can't like get enough air. But usually this thing I can shake.

MR. D: Are these things related, doctor? Is there any similarity between them? I mean aside from the fact that they're different symptoms, but is there a common cause?

DOCTOR: Well, I guess there might be. What common cause would you be looking for?

MR. D: I don't know. From what I've gathered here we all seem to be to a lesser degree—a greater or lesser extent, anticipating the next onslaught, the next occurrence.

DOCTOR: Are you, Mr. E?

MR. E: No.

DOCTOR: Are you, Mr. L?

MR. E: There is no point in it, it's so minute, so fractional, so nonexistent.

MR. L: I hope there isn't.

DOCTOR: Isn't what?

MR. L: Onslaught.

MR. D: Do you look forward to worrying again? I've heard you say you do; you worry about worrying.

MR. L: I hope I won't have to in the future. I keep telling myself I don't.

MR. D: We all hope we won't have to. The thing is whether we do or not.

MR. H: I had an experience yesterday with a relative of mine, for some reason he brought this out, that he doesn't worry about anything, particularly involving the whole idea of time. He doesn't anticipate anything. And almost to the extent where this was wrong, you know. Sometimes he won't know what day it is in the week. (This describes another way of averting anxiety by avoidance. This is the way Mr. D hopes to handle his problems.)

MR. E: I never do.

MR. H: This man has a very responsible job and it doesn't affect him in any way. I just thought I'd mention this. Nothing bothers him, he has a real cool head, he doesn't worry about whether he has to mail a letter tomorrow.

MR. L: How do you know he doesn't? He may just say it.

MR. H: Right. Maybe the fact that he did bring it out, true.

DOCTOR: What do you say, Mr. J? Do you wait to be uncomfortable or anticipate being uncomfortable?

MR. J: Yeah, I guess so.

DOCTOR: Mr. K?

MR. K: The only time I get nervous or anything is when I've done something that I know isn't right. So if I pull a stunt then I'm constantly worrying until I fix it. But I don't worry about the next time I'm going to do something.

DOCTOR: You're suggesting then that their episodes might have some relation to something they feel there is going to be some consequence of, or something like that. (Another attempt to clarify the causes of anxiety.)

MR. K: Something I know there is going to be a consequence to. I mean if I start cutting class a lot or letting something slide, it's going to bother me.

DOCTOR: Do you think Mr. D feels there is going to be some consequence of this heated discussion and starts worrying?

MR. K: Well, I can't say what causes—if something happens and then he worries I think there could be a relation; but worrying if something might happen, I can't see that.

DOCTOR: Mr. E, you seemed interested in saying something.

MR. E: Just then?

DOCTOR: Yeah.

MR. E: No, I just had kind of a momentary attack and I was looking around to see if you noticed. But you hadn't. That's all. (Mr. E refers to his presumed epileptic momentary lapses of consciousness. Although he had three-cycle-per-second spike-dome discharges on the electroencephalogram, the lapses he described could not be positively identified. The occurrence of a lapse at this point in the group discussion suggests a psychogenic episode based on anxiety rather than one on the basis of abnormal brain physiology.)

MR. H: Momentary attack of what? I'm sorry.

MR. E: Well, I don't know, you'll have to ask the doctor.

MR. H: Oh, I see. I thought it was about what we were talking about.

MR. E: Well, it is and it isn't. I mean it's the closest thing that I have in relation to what you're talking about, as far as I can see. I don't think it's really related to anxiety. In a very vague sense, the fantasy connected with this last thing was I was sending medicines to Java.

DOCTOR: Tranquilizers?

MR. E: No.

DOCTOR: That's what they are.

MR. E: Those things, whatever they are.

DOCTOR: Mainly tranquilizers. Different sizes, sorts, shapes, colors.

MR. E: They don't need them in that country. Maybe they do these days. Four battalions moved into the capital yesterday.

DOCTOR: Do you have a job? (This was designed to bring Mr. E back to his everyday problems in living. He appeared to want to discuss his interest in the Far East and via a discussion of the drug samples to talk about things referring to his "special" relationship to the therapist.)

MR. E: Right. And I'm going to change it next week or so for a better one.

DOCTOR: What do you do?

MR. E: Right now it's purely a clerical job through a temporary agency, marking time until I find out from schools and if I find out one way or the other; then I can plan, either get a job or go to school. But I don't want to tell anybody I'm going to school, although this makes it more difficult in looking for a job. It's working with a company I was assigned to at random. It deals with transporting stocks and records into cards and putting little things in envelopes, with a slight variation all day long. The next, probably in a week or so, I'll be working again on a temporary basis into the fall as an airline ticket agent for (an airline).

DOCTOR: Air what?

MR. E: (An airline). (A name)—that's what they call themselves. Their slogan is (a slogan). And that's that for the time being. I rather enjoy it; no problem. And it also kind of sucks me into society. I wasn't quite as hostile as I appeared last week to advertisements, and so forth. I exaggerated to stress the point that it exists. All right, this job gets me into various things, you know, routinization, social security system, and so forth, and so on. I don't really object to this. My father decided to retire two or three weeks ago; I don't know whether I told you. It doesn't really matter, in a sense. In a sense it will change lives around, but that's all. His job is physically too hard for him to handle and he's having attacks in his chest, and so forth, and I guess it amounts to old age. (It is evident that Mr. E thinks of getting a job as putting him into contact with the things most other people encounter also.)

DOCTOR: How old is he?

MR. E: Sixty-seven. And it's all day long. His memory is beginning to slip and his hearing is beginning to go and he is constantly worried about missing an order and then losing a few thousand dollars, or something or other, and not being able to patch it up because everything is fed onto the IBM machine after you finish it. He's very worried. He smokes a lot. He's trying to persuade his partners to hire another man or I mean to have a partnership arrangement with a fourth person. And then they said yes, and then they said no. He hates his partners. It's purely a monetary arrangement. When I say hate, I almost mean it. He will ignore an invitation to the wedding of one of the partner's daughter, so on and so forth. He won't go; he'll send a card. They'll never come to him; he won't go there, which is rather interesting. Anyway, his father and his grandfather are all self-employed. I guess part of this is getting used to the idea. He didn't go into the firm before he was sixty and before that he was self-employed. That may or may not have something to do with it. Very much. You know, his brother won't have anything to do particularly—there is a lot of trouble integrating himself— (Mr. E goes into some of his family background. His unusual family had served to isolate him from his peers.)

DOCTOR: I know this is much news to me, you know, what you say.

MR. E: Well, I don't know whether it's relevant or interesting. I mean, I'm taking up other people's time.

DOCTOR: Well, I think that—

MR. E: I admire his brother and I *have* had much more when I was a child. This is the gentleman who had cancer about two years ago. Architect. He's a bachelor. He's sixty-five. It was through him I came to like classical music, perhaps traveling. This gentleman really has lived for his travels. He's worked a hundred hours a week most of his life and then taken a year off after five years to go to Europe, or some place like that. He's done this two or three times. And in recent years he's had, as a perfectionist, he's had much trouble with his clients. Because if they want to build a colonial style house, he'll want to build one. And they'll say let's put in these doors, it's cheaper, and he'll say that's not colonial. And he's been increasingly unable to work with clients in his later years. So while he had cancer recently and it hasn't helped his nervous system, he'd gotten to this point anyway. Why he's a bachelor, I don't know. There is a very interesting thing there. I don't know what to relate to this at all. There is another sister in my father's family who is also a spinster, lives over here. In the last ten years she has probably spent two at (a psychiatric hospital) for being mentally upset one way or another, I'm not quite sure what the symptoms are and I don't know how to describe the thing. But that's just my father's side of the family. I think it's rather interesting that while my father and his brother are self-employed and then his brother and sister—his sister has never worked and she's a spinster, this is somewhat significant to me anyway. Why I don't know. While this is new to you, have I gotten you confused?

DOCTOR: No.

MR. L: Last week when I left here, I was thinking on the train of starting a diary of some sort, just writing down what I do every day and how I spend my time and what I think about. And then I thought it wouldn't be such a good idea because if I constantly look back on the days, I might get more depressed if I didn't improve. And if I did I'd get my hopes up too high. So I didn't. I didn't do it.

MR. H: What's wrong with getting your hopes up too high?

MR. E: I missed a phrase there. Your hopes up to high about what?

MR. L: Recovering, changing. I'm trying not to let things excite me. I'm trying to be calm.

MR. E: You know, you have a mixture of two things, sort of a fatalism and a hyperactivity or a hyperconcern or active concern. And these things I think are valuable in any person. You have to be fatalistic about things, spilt milk; you just have to say, well, that's that. I tend to think sometimes your're fatalistic and concerned about the wrong things; you just switch them around; it's just a question of arrangement. It's easy to say that.

MR. L: You're right, that's what I was thinking too.

MR. E: Sort of like there is two things in a painting, basically color and form, and you're all kinds of colors but not too much form.

MR. L: I'm trying to do things that relax me. I mean a lot of times I noticed before I'd feel sort of guilty about having a good time because I'd think, well, I should be doing something else or I'm not getting any real constructive benefit out of it. But now I have a different view. I'm trying to do, you know, as much as I can to enjoy myself. I'm not—you know, I think of consequences. I don't go overboard and just enjoy myself all the time, but I try to do as much as I can, reasonably can. Like this morning I was a little depressed. I don't remember about what. And I didn't have a class till two. And it looked like a nice day so I went to Central Park and I went ice skating. That always seems to relax me, the organ music and you skate in time to the music. It's very relaxing. And I was enjoying that for awhile until I made a—I tried to pick up a few girls and I was a little disappointed, so that made me a little unhappy, but I wasn't that unhappy. I had a good time.

Mr. E: Well, were these girls good skaters?

Mr. L: I must have tried about three or four. They weren't bad.

Mr. E: What, as girls—

Mr. L: Both ways. One was a married woman. I didn't realize it. She had a glove on and she took off her left glove and flashes her ring in front of me. The old men there were having more luck than I was. There was one old fellow about sixty-five. He's going over to every young girl he sees, he was as lively as anything.

Mr. D: Maybe it was the paternal attitude that they liked.

Mr. L: It wasn't. Maybe he tried to get away with it that way, I don't know. He tried the younger women, then he tried the older women. He was doing pretty well. He was doing better than I was.

Mr. E: I remember seeing an old couple once, probably nearly seventy, making out in the back of a bus, and I thought what a great thing for love to last that long. (Almost no expression of warm positive feelings between members of Mr. E's family were known. He longed for affection, yet had been conditioned against physical demonstrativeness.)

* * *

Mr. H: Didn't you say at one time that when the chips were really down you really came through?

Mr. L: If you're really down, yeah, I'll force myself to work. (The degree that Mr. L allows himself to be disabled by his symptoms is shown to be unnecessary. That he can help himself if he tries becomes apparent.)

Mr. D: But this is no way to carry on. We all, I think, are able to do that when we concentrate.

Mr. L: Not everybody.

Mr. D: At least I am, let's say. But one can't go on through an entire day of being occupied and working just to take one's mind off it.

Mr. L: No, I'm not doing that.

Mr. E: Don't you feel the chips are down every day?

Mr. H: No, the idea that he forces himself he's able to overcome.

Mr. D: Yeah, but the forcing was being actively engaged in something.

Mr. H: All right, think of it that way.

Mr. D: But you can't do it twenty-four hours a day.

Mr. L: It's very difficult for me to do that, to force myself to do something to forget about something else, because then I get twice as bad.

Mr. H: I should think just the fact that you want to overcome it should be that much of a motivation. (The relationship between motivation to improve and the secondary gain of the symptoms is alluded to but not taken up.)

Mr. D: During the course of a work day I find there are some days that in the course of a job I'll be occupied the entire day; then there are other times when the work is developing that I'll have nothing to do. And it's at those times that I have nothing to do that—

Mr. H: Where you're most vulnerable.

Mr. D: Exactly. Where I think about myself, where I think about my problems.

Mr. H: Don't you find there are times in spite of the fact you have nothing to do you can think about yourself and it won't bother you?

Mr. D: Sure.

MR. H: Yet there are times when you are busy—

MR. D: Absolutely. There is no set formula. You can't say it's going to happen such and such a way. The only thing I can say is when I get into these animated discussions it usually does happen after that. And it isn't that I don't enjoy the discussions; I rather like that.

MR. H: You mean the after effects.

MR. D: Yeah.

MR. E: I find a certain benefit from these discussions because it's more easy for me to observe the actions I am participating in and evaluate them. One's more conscious of behavior. (This is one of the benefits expected from the group psychotherapy. Mr. E knows this and being a compliant person says it to the therapist, really. The positive transference aspect of this is obvious. Mr. E has been able to perform better at school and to go to work at a regular job with the help of his treatment. The negative part of his transference feelings soon becomes apparent in his arranging to miss some of his appointments.)

MR. D: Your own or others?

MR. E: Both. It's less action and reaction rather than calculated action. That's all. I hope you aren't disturbed about this. Are you jealous because I'm going to work for the airline?

DOCTOR: Why should I be jealous?

MR. E: Because you said, "You better not, you better come here; arrange for a job so you can come here."

DOCTOR: Yeah. It's important that you try to continue your appointments here.

MR. E: You think so?

DOCTOR: Yeah.

MR. E: Well—all right.

DOCTOR: I mean, I don't know what you can do about the job. Maybe you can't do anything about it, maybe you can.

MR. E: You see, this is the only way I can possibly pay for them. It's sort of ironic.

MR. L: Well, he has a session on Thursday afternoon too, so if you get shifts you can work it into one or the other.

MR. E: Well, the shifts vary from week to week and I'm not

sure what they are. They go up through twelve o'clock at night at the latest and they start at eight in the morning, eight or nine at the earliest. The days one gets off every week vary from week to week.

Mr. L: Do you find that interesting, changing your schedule around?

Mr. E: I couldn't care less. I'd work at any given period during the day. It doesn't bother me, I can sleep at any time.

Mr. L: I find that more interesting. I couldn't stand going to school the same time every day and getting out the same time. I really couldn't stand it.

Mr. E: Well, there is a certain security in routine.

Mr. L: I hate it. I hate when I go to work because I go in at nine and I get out at five, the same thing every day, eat from twelve to one.

Mr. E: You don't have to eat.

Mr. L: No.

Mr. E: Let it go. Do something.

Mr. L: I get hungry. The high point in the day.

Mr. E: Yeah, but it's good, you know.

Mr. L: What?

Mr. E: It's a way of seeing how you can practice self-discipline.

Mr. L: You're forced into sitting behind that desk all day.

Mr. E: That's one way. There are positive and negative aspects to this, denial.

Mr. L: I do that enough by myself. I want to go in the opposite direction. I can only indulge in one thing, make myself a wreck.

Mr. E: What kind of a wreck?

Mr. L: So I can't function the way I want to. It's amazing. Some days when I feel down in the dumps everything is disgusting, everything looks disgusting to me, anything just annoys me, people annoy me, places annoy me, the school annoys me. Then when I'm in a good mood it just seems like they aren't the same things really. The subway seems great, and I listen to the noises in the subway; I look at the people, everyone seems great. That's not too often. I'd like it to be more often. I get more out of things. It's amazing how much you can get out of things if you let yourself, if you put something into it. (Mr. L has learned to get more satisfactions during the course of his treatment.)

MR. D: Can you do that more often than you have been?

MR. L: I'm trying to do it more often. I just feel I've denied myself too much from life.

MR. D: Well, I think you've got a lot of life ahead of you yet.

MR. L: Well, I don't know.

MR. E: Well, it's slipping out.

MR. D: What is?

MR. E: Life. It gets shorter every day. If he doesn't put any—

MR. D: If he tries too hard it's no good either.

MR. E: He mustn't feel he's in a desperate situation.

MR. L: I remember through high school I never had any hobbies and during the weekend I'd usually work. I would hardly even go out—not work, just go through the motions. I'd stay in the house a lot and I didn't let myself do anything I really wanted to. Now I'm doing more things that I always wanted to do. (Mr. L has become less fearful and less rigid.)

MR. D: Doesn't that make you feel better in yourself, the knowledge that you're doing it?

MR. L: It does.

MR. D: So you are coming along.

MR. L: Yeah. I feel that's very important and it's helped me.

MR. D: So the picture isn't as bleak as you painted it. You are making progress.

MR. L: I don't know if I am.

MR. D: Well, you just said you are.

MR. L: Maybe.

DOCTOR: Why would somebody complain about not making progress even though at the same time he would say that he'd done it, that he had improved, made some progress? (To call attention to Mr. L's progress and ambivalence.)

MR. D: Well, I would hardly want to put my person in your chair but in my own opinion, and not based on any medical knowledge whatsoever, it seems it's a very self-defeating attitude that he has. He doesn't give himself a chance to attempt anything. If he does attempt anything he has already prejudged it with failure and if he does lessen the element of thinking that he's going to fail if he should even in the slightest way not succeed in his undertaking, he thoroughly dooms himself.

DOCTOR: Why do you think he would do that?

MR. D: Why?

DOCTOR: Yeah.

MR. D: I don't know. There might be a certain gratification even in the failing; the idea that I've predicted I'm going to fail and I was right when I did fail, the prediction came true.

MR. E: Or the thought that he's never really tried might be comforting, you know.

MR. D: What would you say, doctor?

DOCTOR: Well, you don't agree with Mr. E?

MR. D: No.

MR. E: I can reverse that around by saying—well, never mind.

MR. D: Of course, in what I've said I might be reflecting some of my own thinking, and Mr. E on the other hand might be giving you his particular slant on the thing. In other words, I'm reading possibly some of my own symptoms into Mr. L and that's why I can't see Mr. E's point. (Here he begins to take what he said about Mr. L and apply it to himself. In group psychotherapy this applying of comments about the others to oneself occurs frequently. This encourages self-understanding in both the speaker and the one spoken about.)

DOCTOR: Uh-huh.

MR. E: I can't see much difference in them really. I just said the same thing turned around.

DOCTOR: Well, turned around another way, "Well, I'm going to do it, but I don't want anybody to know it," or "I'm afraid to learn about it myself; let's not and say we did," which is the other way around, or "I'm getting better but I better not admit it," or something like that. (The positive transference reaction involved in the patient's telling the doctor he is better must be correlated with the reality of his improvement. The fear of objection to success or improved status can occur on a transference basis also.)

Mr. D: Uh-huh. In other words, it's self-punishment.

Doctor: Do you think that's what it is?

Mr. H: I wonder about that, whether I'm not just punishing myself along the same lines as you are (indicating Mr. L).

Doctor: Self-punishment?

Mr. H: Yeah.

Doctor: For what? (This was a way of asking the patients to examine their feelings of guilt. Their irrational guilt acted to inhibit their effectiveness at times.)

Mr. H: I don't know.

Doctor: I've got a bunch of crooks or criminals here that need to be punished? What is this?

Mr. L: Maybe I feel I don't have the ability to accomplish something like this.

Mr. K: Like what? You lost me.

Mr. L: By snapping out of thinking the way I do.

Mr. E: You don't have any confidence in yourself? in your intelligence? your masculinity?

Mr. L: I don't know.

Mr. D: I myself know I suffer from a lack of a degree of self-confidence.

Mr. L: Because I haven't really accomplished anything.

Mr. E: A lack of pride?

Mr. L: Yeah. I just haven't done very much. Every time I try to do something I let myself down. I disappoint myself every time I get over-worried about something. I say I'm not going to do it and I do it. It's a big disappointment when I offer myself to someone and they just turn me down and turn away from me and it's repeatedly done; it's a big disappointment.

Mr. D: You see, I've never met with that—most of the undertakings that I've attempted, although I felt they wouldn't come off, have usually come off quite well. But this hasn't lessened my apprehension that they won't, up to a point. I find after I made the same mistake of anticipating things will come off and they don't, I write them off.

MR. E: Of course, this has to do with what you try.

MR. D: Naturally.

MR. E: You might be attempting something that's too easy for you.

MR. D: No, I don't feel that the undertakings are that easy. If I felt that they were that easy I wouldn't be worrying about the outcome.

MR. E: No, if you were the worrying kind you might even take an easier thing than you can do. I don't know.

MR. L: When things go wrong, like when I fail, or I don't succeed in something, I sort of make it like it's beyond my control or it's like a dream, it's not really happening. Sometimes I do that, I guess, to try to avoid hurting myself. I remember when I was younger, especially in junior high school, I think that's when I started getting nervous; I think it was in junior high school. I had a teacher for the seventh grade and she was a real old-fashioned type of teacher, about fifty-five years old; she was probably still a virgin, and she kept me in every day after three for some reason. I don't know what she was trying to do to me really. She'd talk to me every afternoon and tell me more or less what a rotten person I was; I had no control, I was talking all the time—I wasn't even doing these things—I had no sense of responsibility, I had nothing. I don't know. I don't know why she did it. Then she called my mother to school once, I remember, and she started screaming at me and then my mother started yelling at her, "What are you yelling at my son like that for? He has so much ability." It's the first time she said I had ability. "And he's just wasting his life, he's just wasting everything. Look at his assignment book, what a mess it is." And she tore it up. And I was getting very nervous, very sensitive at that age. And then I had another beauty in the ninth grade, same type of teacher, and I had to sit in front of her, first row. Oh, she hated me.

MR. H: You must have been a bad kid in school.

MR. L: I wasn't. I didn't do a darn thing. I sat there and minded my own business and these old bags would always pick on me. She made me so frightened. I was afraid every time I went into that class. She would always embarrass me. She'd call me uncouth; she'd call me everything. (This catharsis of feelings about teachers and his mother is also an exposition of material Mr. L and the others can examine.)

MR. H: For no reason?

MR. L: Not for anything that I saw. I didn't do anything terrible.

MR. E: Your—did your parents have to use strong discipline, or was a word or two enough?

MR. L: They never really disciplined me.

MR. E: I mean are you very sensitive to criticism?

MR. L: Yeah.

MR. E: So physical punishment might not have been necessary, very rarely.

MR. L: I was always very obstinate; I was always obstinate. I was spoiled when I was young. If I wanted something, if I put up enough fuss I would get it. I can still remember when I was little they'd tell me to do one thing, I'd do something else. I always felt that way about authority. Yet, you know, in school I conformed. When they told me to do something I did it. But I know at home I felt if I listened to my parents I'd be subservient; or anybody really, I wouldn't want to listen to anybody. They'd tell me to do something, I wouldn't want to do it. I wouldn't join a camp because that was one of the reasons. (This may be related to some of Mr. L's negative transference reactions.)

MR. D: And none of this carried over into school? In school you weren't that way?

MR. L: No, in school I was always described as quiet. I'd take orders. You know, I was never a troublemaker.

MR. E: Did you look forward to going to school?

MR. L: No. When I was young I was scared stiff of it. Maybe because of some of the teachers—no, it wasn't, because in public school I was deathly afraid. Maybe it was just something I couldn't control.

MR. E: Did your parents ever let you stay home because of this?

MR. L: No. Well, sometimes they did, yes, once in awhile. But I went. I mean I had to go so I went. I was always frightened. All my life I have been frightened of things. Now I think back when I was young, there is a lot of times I find myself wishing I was young again so I wouldn't think of the things I'm thinking of now. Then I think when I was young I was still miserable. I was always—I was always miserable. I was never really happy. I was looking through my album; my parents kept an album of me each year as I grew up. It was all right when I was very young, but then I noticed when I reached about five, a lot of times, you know, I'd have a sour look on my face, very annoyed. I never really had too many friends, I remember when I was younger. I was alone most of the time, do things myself. I don't know if it was because I didn't like groups or I felt that they would just ignore me or I was afraid of them; I don't know what it was. Still I don't like groups of people. I don't like to mingle in. I always noticed that I complain a lot about anything really. If I'm very hot sometimes it becomes really unbearable to me. Or if things aren't just so, I'm always complaining about things. Not always, but, you know, once in awhile. I do it too often, I think, a little too much. If I don't get something exactly the way I want it I get very, very, very annoyed. Like I was supposed to see this girl I'm going with yesterday; I was supposed to see her in the morning, and then she had to go to—her father works in a shoe store and his boss has another one in (another town), a ladies' shoe store. So she went with him to get shoes and I was going to go with her. But then the father said, you know, I shouldn't come, too many people in the store. So I said all right. So then she said she'd call me when she got home. She didn't call. I figured she'd call about two. She didn't call until four. All day long I was saying—I was waiting, you know, and she said, "I'm too tired now; I'm knocked out. I don't think I can see you today." And I just get very, very annoyed. It's like I got so annoyed, it was like she was telling me she'll never see me again. I could even compare it to that. It just didn't go the way I wanted it to.

Mr. E: Do you think you can get along without her?

Mr. L: I don't know. I think I'd have a lot of trouble.

Mr. E: Do you think you're overly dependent on the relationship?

Mr. L: I might be. That's why I'm trying to go out more.

But I don't seem to be succeeding. And every time I go out I get more depressed. I don't know, I used to have more success than I do now. I don't know what to do about it. I'm trying to be myself, I don't know, the self I want to be. I don't know. It's mysterious to me; it's like I have a hex on me.

DOCTOR: Shall we stop?

* * *

Some Observations of Session 3

As the group work begins to affect him, Mr. E says, "I find a certain benefit from these discussions because it's more easy for me to observe the actions I am participating in and evaluate them. One's more conscious of behavior." This is picked up by Mr. L. Mr. E then brings out his resistance to treatment by speaking of it in terms of a time conflict with his working hours.

Again day-to-day things were discussed with regard to feelings and mental operations.

Mr. L became anxious to do something about his way of approaching everyday problems.

Messrs. D, E, and H questioned their ways of thinking.

Mr. L joined the discussion and compared himself to them.

Unwittingly he carried this on and discussed his feelings toward a girl he wants to date.

He wound up by saying he was a failure with a hex on him so far as girls are concerned now.

In this session much self-exploration and self-observation have occurred. The patients have compared themselves with one another, then each has reflected on himself in terms of the ideas developed in the group discussion.

Note Concerning
Verbatim Excerpts, Comments, and Observations

The verbatim excerpts have a high degree of accuracy for the verbal content of the portions of the group psychotherapy sessions presented in this way. As anyone who has had experience with attempts to record and reproduce the content of psychotherapy sessions knows, it is almost impossible to obtain a complete record. The records are necessarily incomplete because of the inflections of the voices, the nonverbal communications, and the inadvertent and adventitious material that cannot always be correlated with the group psychotherapy is not easily recorded.

The parenthetical comments about the transcripts and the other notes and observations concerning them are fragmentary. No attempt has been made to be complete. A complete presentation of all the aspects of each exchange would fill many volumes.

The overdetermined nature of each speech by the therapist as well as each line from the patients could lead to an almost infinite number of interpretations. Those provided in this book are not intended to be complete but to give a representative sample of the interpretations possible.

The reader should also be aware that the interest and stimulation of the actual psychotherapy sessions are difficult to evoke in the transcript.

Chapter 10

A PATIENT LEAVES THE GROUP

When a patient who has been treated with group psychotherapy has improved his general functioning to the point where treatment no longer seems necessary, he should be discharged. At times a patient will decide for himself that he is getting along well enough to try things on his own. The therapist is aware of the general state of adjustment of his patients from their talk in the group and by his direct inquiries. Before the patient raises the question about discontinuing treatment, the therapist should have considered the possibility and mentioned it to him.

Saying to a patient that he appears to be getting along well and that he should consider how much longer treatment should continue precipitates a self-evaluation. This is often anxiety-provoking. His reaction shows the reality orientation of the patient. Realistically, patients come to be treated and ultimately discharged.

Some patients must return after discharge for further treatment. For still others, their regular treatment visits of once a week for one and one-half hours in group psychotherapy can be reduced to one visit a month or even less frequently.

Groups in which the same patients remain for several years without change are probably not therapeutic. Such groups may serve a social or mutually sustaining function, but do not make for constructive individual change. Unavoidably, therapeutic groups suffer casualties. Change is always accompanied by stress; at times it is beyond the tolerance of a patient and he drops out.

Patients who cannot tolerate group psychotherapy, regardless of their being seemingly well-suited for this kind of treatment, should be permitted to leave the group. Individual appointments aimed at attempting to understand the difficulty should be arranged for them.

Occasionally, patients threaten to discontinue treatment to coerce the therapist into giving them more individual attention. Although the therapist should be liberal in arranging individual appointments, he must not allow a patient to subvert the group by using individual sessions with the therapist to avoid therapeutic work in the group.

Some patients who can neither work in the group nor use individual treatment as an ancillary should be discharged with the proviso that treatment may be better suited for them at some future date. Such patients may be referred to another psychiatrist for consultation or perhaps another style of treatment. It is very important that departing patients understand that their being discharged from the group does not preclude future treatment efforts by the same or another therapist.

Patients who have to discontinue treatment because of external circumstances, such as their going to another state to take a job, a sudden death in the family, or other personal catastrophe should be given every consideration in arranging to terminate treatment and find some kind of help elsewhere.

Mrs. G had been in group psychotherapy for two years. She was a compulsive personality who had had episodes of anxiety and depression partly related to her husband's increasing prominence in local political and professional organizations. Initially, she was hospitalized; after her discharge, she was treated by medication and individual psychotherapy.

During her first year of treatment, she had had to be hospitalized three times for periods of less than two weeks each. In the second year of her treatment she was started in group psychotherapy which became her primary treatment, although individual interviews and medication were continued. During her third year of treatment, her anxiety diminished and she was able to move about more freely and to resume many of the activities she had given up when she was most uncomfortable. Her circumscribed, ritualistic, tightly organized style of living became somewhat relaxed.

Although a bright college graduate in chemistry, she had worked as an executive secretary, but had never read newspapers. During her treatment, she became much more aware of the interests and activities of other people and less concerned with her own approach to life.

During the last five months of group psychotherapy, her medication was gradually reduced and she remained comfortable most of the time. In the group, she functioned more appropriately and was not so constrained to silence by anxiety, nor provoked to outbursts when she was unable to control the tensions evoked by the group discussions. Her behavior in the group became spontaneous and more relevant intellectually and emotionally. It became apparent that she no longer needed group psychotherapy.

Two months before she discontinued this treatment, she was told in a group session that she appeared to be getting along very well and that she did not appear to need to come to the group meetings every week.

Her response was that she would rather stop altogether than to come every two weeks or once a month. During her period of treatment in group psychotherapy, the spacing out of visits had been a prelude to termination for other patients who had improved. Two weeks before her discharge, she said on her arrival at a group session that she felt she did not need to come any longer, that she would come the next week and then no more. This was permitted.

Contact with Mrs. G one year later, when she came to have a Motor Vehicle Bureau form filled out (required because she had been hospitalized for mental illness), and a conversation with her husband on that occasion revealed that she had maintained her more comfortable and more flexible way of getting along.

Miss C, a remitted stuperous catatonic schizophrenic woman, who has been described before, had been treated since her initial catatonic episode six years previously. She had received electric shock treatments and had been hospitalized for about six weeks, during which time she improved on Thorazine. Subsequently, she had been treated in individual psychotherapy for eleven months and then had started in group and individual psychotherapy. Group psychotherapy had been her primary treatment for four and a half years.

She had been employed steadily for the past five years, at

first in a routine stereotyped clerical job. She was presently working as a card punch machine operator, punching cards for computerized payroll calculators. Miss C led a quiet life, living at home with her parents, going to work regularly, and attending group psychotherapy sessions once a week for one and one-half hours. She had taken no medication for the past four years. Occasional individual appointments had had to be arranged when she became upset about the amorous, incestuous overtures made by her alcoholic brother, and on one occasion when a visit to a dentist she had not known previously had been accompanied by his quizzing her about her social and love life.

When Miss C saw Mrs. G leave the group, she remarked, in one group session, "You know, doctor, I have been in treatment for a long time and I have seen a lot of people get better and leave the group. I wonder if I am ever going to be able to come less frequently and ever be discharged." The therapist replied, "That is an important thing to consider. This group should have a beginning, a middle, and an end. You are right. Suppose we try it with your coming once every two weeks rather than every week for awhile and see how it goes."

When Miss C returned the following week, she was visibly perturbed and said she was not sure she should leave the group so suddenly. The therapist reassured her, saying that it was perfectly all right. She was also reassured by other members of the group.

She was advised to come less frequently unless something particular came up to disturb her. Miss C was pacified, and began coming once every two weeks and eventually once every four weeks. The therapist would never completely withdraw from contact with this patient.

Chapter 11

THE THERAPIST LEAVES THE GROUP

In institutional settings and in most private practice, the group psychotherapist will know his schedule several months in advance. If he must stop treating the group, he must tell the patients so as far in advance as possible and also let them know the definite date as soon as it has been fixed. This gives the patients an opportunity to work out some of their emotional reactions to the therapist and his leaving them, as well as providing them with an opportunity to prepare themselves for other treatment arrangements.

When the group psychotherapist cannot arrange to attend a group meeting, he should notify the patients as far in advance as possible. If that is not possible, someone at the place where the group would ordinarily meet should be advised to tell the patients the meeting has been postponed and, if possible, when the next session is scheduled. If this cannot be done, patients should be told they will be notified later. This is extremely important.

When there is a change of therapists in teaching settings, the prospective new group psychotherapist should attend the group as an observer as many sessions as possible in advance of his becoming the therapist. He should be introduced to the group but should not participate in the treatment as therapist until the therapist he is replacing has left the group.

The prospective group psychotherapist should also attend the supervisory sessions for his group with the psychotherapist he is to replace. He should discuss the reactions of the group with him and the supervisor at every opportunity.

Most of the time at the beginning of his work with an established and working group, the new psychotherapist will get the negative feelings of its members toward the former therapist.

He will hear complaints about the change in therapists and about the youth and inexperience of therapists. He should be aware of the meaning of this kind of talk. If he listens carefully, he will often be able to relate it to past experiences the patients have had with others in a caretaker position to them. Often in carrying the ideas of one patient to the other patients for their opinions of these ideas, the patients will make comparisons to previous treatment and to social and family situations that have been important to them. The complaints directed at the new therapist have only a small kernel of reality. Knowing this, he can undertake the treatment with more assurance.

A second-year resident, who was to begin treating a group on the first of July joined it in May as an observer. He sat quietly at one side of the room, avoiding a prominent role in the group meetings. The group response to his presence varied according to the reality situation and the psychodynamics of the patients. A patient or two with impulsive makeup directed questions at him. When he did not answer, the conductor of the group said, "Dr. R really cannot answer you. I wonder why you ask."

The therapist explained that the observer would sit with the group but would not participate in the sessions until the first of July, when he would be the psychotherapist in charge. Many complaints about "changing doctors all the time" and about having young, inexperienced doctors occurred after the first of July. Some of these had come up between May and July. Expressions of gratitude and good wishes for the future were also expressed to the therapist who had been treating the group for the past year.

Chapter 12

SUMMARY

Utilizing as its principal mechanism the salutary effect of the microsociety of the psychotherapy group on the personality organization of each individual in the group, this treatment is indicated for patients with disorders in which their personality is distorted or poorly integrated. This includes the bulk of patients who apply for outpatient treatment. From the psychoanalytic viewpoint group psychotherapy is related to the thesis that the style of the ego or character is socially determined.*

The comparisons that patients in group psychotherapy make with one another serve to promote self-evaluation as well as to provide a variety of solutions to common problems from different viewpoints. Personality distortions are pointed out and alternate modes of behavior are offered. Impoverishment of adaptive social devices is overcome through the tonic of many contributions that each member receives from the group.

The healthy core or, at times, residue of social and intrapsychic machinery varies from patient to patient. Patients with similar defects see them in one another and are able to learn better ways of living from one another.

Group psychotherapy helps patients with a wide range of psychiatric disorders but does not preclude other kinds of treatments. Combinations of group and individual psychotherapy are useful for many patients, and various somatic treatments are possible during the course of group psychotherapy. Many patients can be treated effectively with group psychotherapy whose economic capability has been impaired by one of the more severe mental disorders. For persons with such disorders it provides a kind of adequate treatment that is likely to be within their means.

Patients selected for group psychotherapy are those whose

---

* Fenichel, O. *op. cit.*

severe symptoms have been borne somehow by the patient previously. The treatment supports him in carrying his burden and ultimately makes it lighter by relieving him of some of the trouble.

Psychiatrists who practice group psychotherapy should be trained to provide this kind of treatment. The training essentials are observation of a working psychotherapy group and adequate supervision in conducting such groups.

Patients are selected for group psychotherapy because they have an affliction of the personality organization itself. Some patients with personality disorders and others who are remitted psychotics have managed to tolerate symptoms because there is a core or residue of healthy function that can be increased by the addition of contributions from other patients in the group. These patients have to be selected on this basis and prepared for group psychotherapy, just as they have to be oriented to any other kind of medical treatment.

At first the new patient in the group is afraid and curious. Part of the therapist's task is to help the patient work out these reactions in the group. The reactions of the individuals in the group to new patients embody their established patterns of meeting newcomers. The therapist utilizes the verbalizations or other communications of group members to a new patient as part of the treatment.

Patients leave the group when they no longer need its help and for other reasons. Patients who are severely and/or chronically ill need to be able to get group treatment intermittently. For this reason, it is essential to have open groups that new patients are free to enter and leave voluntarily.

The treatment of patients in group psychotherapy is terminated like any medical treatment. The patient who improves may have the frequency of his visits reduced or he may stop abruptly when he is ready. Treatment failures should be recognized at the earliest opportunity, and the patient should thereupon be assisted in making other arrangements. Patients who are going to require care indefinitely should be recognized and treated accordingly.

When the psychotherapist leaves a group its members must be notified as far in advance as possible. Patients need to know that subsequent treatment can be arranged for them if and when it becomes necessary.

Examples of the phenomena of group psychotherapy have been illustrated by the verbatim excerpts. Notes, observations, and comments on these verbatim reports have been provided.

Group psychotherapy has established a tradition of worthwhile treatment. Its theory is hampered by our lack of a scientific psychology, yet we have a body of knowledge that provides a practical treatment technique from which further useful theory can be derived.

SELECTED BIBLIOGRAPHY

The following publications are recommended for further reading:

Berne, E.: *Transactional Analysis in Psychotherapy.* New York, Grove, 1961.

Foulkes, S. H.: *Therapeutic Group Analysis.* New York, Int. Univs., 1965.

Freeman, T., Cameron, J. L., and McGhie, A.: *Chronic Schizophrenia.* New York, Int. Univs., 1958.

Johnson, J. A., Jr.: *Group Therapy: A Practical Approach.* New York, McGraw, 1963.

Klapman, J. W.: *Group Psychotherapy Theory and Practice,* 2nd ed. New York, Grune, 1959.

Mullin, H., and Rosenbaum, M.: *Group Psychotherapy Theory and Practice.* New York, Free Press of Glencoe (Macmillan), 1963.

Slavson, S. R.: *An Introduction to Group Therapy.* New York, Commonwealth Fund, 1943.

Wolf, A.: The psychoanalysis of groups. *Amer. J. Psychother., 3*:(No. 4), October, 1949; *4*:(No. 1), January, 1950.

INDEX